Watering th

BETTINA RAE

DEDICATION

For my 3 little stars in the sky.

CONTENTS

ACKNOWLEDGMENTS

I would like to express my deep gratitude to the women in my community, both online and off. Whether directly or indirectly, *you* are the reason this book exists.

To those who contributed their stories, thank you for being so generous and brave. To those who reached out privately when I shared the news of each of my losses, you have helped me in ways I can't even begin to thank you for.

To Andrew; thank you for loving me through the hardest of days and for not letting me give up on our vision for our family.

Finally to my three boys; thank you for always reminding me to keep looking for the light.

INTRODUCTION

"It's your grief my darling and fuck anyone who wants to tell you how to do it" - Geraldine Proudman in Offspring.

Welcome to the shittiest club that you never asked to be a part of. Grieving for a baby lost in your womb is inexplicable to anyone who has not felt it. You will feel lost and broken. Lonely and angry. Heartbroken and desperate longing for your baby.

What helped me the most when I was in the thick of grief was hearing stories of what other women had been through and how they felt. While it didn't stop the pain, it helped me feel a little less alone knowing others had done it before me and survived to find the light again. It made me feel like maybe if they could endure this, then I could too.

The most overwhelming feeling I've felt in this whole process has been feeling lost to grief. My lowest points were those when I was unable to see the way out. When I could no longer see how I could possibly keep living with the grief I felt, and when I was unable to imagine a life where the immense pain of losing my babies would ever fade.

These times were my darkest. I've felt like giving up. I've spent hours desperately searching for an answer to stop the pain. I've ugly cried and screamed and felt unable to get out of bed. Maybe you've had these moments too?

I hope that in these moments, this book can be a comfort to you. I hope my words (and those of the other women who share in this book) might hold your hand and your heart through your darkest places.

I honestly never thought this would be my story. Though of course losing a baby is one of those things that no one *expects* to happen to them.

We know it happens, of course. To friends of friends, to Aunties, to cousins, to sisters, to *other people*. We never imagine it will happen to us. We know the statistics, we just never expect we will *be* the statistic. For some reason our brains forget that someone has to be. Even after you experience it once, you don't expect to luck out again and experience it multiple times over.

I battled with *why* for over a year. Why us? Why our babies? Why now? Why our family? And all the other fun variations of Why. What did we do wrong? What's wrong with my body What did we do to deserve this?'

Why? Why!? WHY?!

The constant questioning is exhausting. It's all-consuming. It sucks all of the joy out of life. It makes connecting with other people, even your partner, extremely difficult.

It makes so much of your life before losing your baby and what you worried about then, feel insignificant and incredibly unnecessary. At the same time it makes other parts of your life feel insurmountable, too big and too scary to get through.

After our three losses in 2016 and early 2017, I found myself in a very dark place. I'd never felt more alone in my life. Despite our best efforts to be there for each other, our individual battles with grief took Andrew (my husband) and I on very different roads and at one point I could no longer see where they came back together.

We both knew after our 3rd loss that we would not be trying again in a hurry. *Perhaps not ever.* He, because he couldn't imagine having to watch me go through it all again. Me, because I knew that some, if not all of the problem was my highly anxious state.

I knew if I were to try again straight away, it would nearly certainly end in another loss. I carried a heavy stone of guilt in my belly about losing our babies and although a part of me could understand that I didn't do anything wrong, I also held onto that guilt like a cross to bear.

It felt like I'd completely forgotten how to enjoy the life I already had, because I was so focused on trying to bring a new life into our family. Of course, I was grateful for my two healthy boys. I was grateful that Andrew had been by my side through all of it. *But I wasn't connected to any of it.* In my heart and head I was too busy battling my own grief demons to enjoy how blessed I already was.

After our 3rd loss a wise woman reached out to remind me that **I needed to start watering the flowers of my life and not just the weeds.** I was already thinking it was time for me to shift my focus onto finding joy again and this message felt like confirmation from the universe.

I needed to teach myself how to live without another baby. I needed to be okay with the fact that there might never be another baby for us. I wasn't entirely giving up, but I did need to give myself a break from it all. I needed time to find myself and the light again.

Within this book I share my journey through grief with you. I hope to show you that there is a way out, not necessarily by having another baby, but by watering the flowers you already have.

This book is not the words of someone who has passed through grief and is now talking to you from the other side (as many of the books on baby loss seem to be.) I wrote these words on some of my darkness days.

I've read too many books on grief and loss that have been written from a very resolved place. From authors who had already made peace with their losses. But I wanted to read the words of someone who was in the same place I was. Not someone who would tell me that time would heal my wounds (even if that were the truth).

When you're still feeling the intense pain of a fresh loss it is extremely hard to hear this perspective. While I could appreciate that maybe one day I would be able to look back and feel this way too, at the time I wanted words that spoke of how they felt *during* the process of healing, not after it had already happened.

I needed raw honesty. I wanted to read my own emotions on a page. I wanted words that mirrored how to be as sad as I was, without feeling like I should be coping 'better' or be more grateful for what I already had.

So I started writing from that place. When I started I didn't know what the ending of this book would look like. Nor did I know how long it would take for me to get there.

While this book is about grief and my personal journey through it, I hope that it is also a story of great love, of finding joy and of hope. I can't always feel all of these things, but I am certainly always looking for them. I want to encourage you to do the same. Even in your darkest moments, keep watering the flowers of your life.

Let me be clear though, this is not a book about overcoming grief. I'm not even sure I believe that's possible anymore. From the many women I've spoken to, some whose losses were over forty years ago, losing a baby is not something you ever completely overcome.

Instead we have to find a way to reconcile the loss within us. It becomes a part of our story and we get to decide what meaning our loss takes on for us long term. It's about finding a way to hold both love and sadness within us at the same time.

This book is for those of you still in the darkness. For those who feel lost and lonely within the transition of loss. It's for you who is in the most excruciating pain you'd never imagined, for those who feel numb to it and for those who aren't really sure how to feel.

Let this book be your guide home. Let it help you find your way again. Let it help you to start putting the broken pieces of yourself back together. No, they won't ever come back in completely the same way as before. You will be forever changed, but I think that too can be a good thing *(eventually)*.

Right now, you might find yourself wishing you could go back to before, when you were naive to it all. Where the world was not such a scary and painful place. But the reality is, this new place, this new way of being in the world, *is also in part about creating you.*

This experience will change you into the person you need to be.
You will see the world in a completely new way.
Your perspective will forever be changed.
You will be know with absolute clarity what is important in your life and what is not.
Everything meaningless will drop away.
Eventually you may even be able to see this new version of yourself as a better one than before.

Though of course, it won't feel like this in the beginning.

In the beginning, it will all just feel *fucking unfair.* You will find yourself muttering or crying out loud that *'This is so unfair!'*

You may even feel like you don't want to go on. But you can. And you will. And you need to go on. Because if you allow yourself to go through the grief, if you can allow yourself to embrace your new reality (however reluctantly) you will discover that grief also brings us gifts.

Strength. Perspective. Bravery. Connection. Empathy.

A new way of being in the world that is fully present to all of it. The good. The bad. The ugly. The painful. The joy *and the despair.*

While it's not all going to be good, having your eyes fully open to life is a powerful new way to experience it.

I will warn you though, the journey to this new place might be a long one. You may find yourself taking one step forward and five steps back. You may catch yourself numbing the pain rather then dealing with it. You may at some point (or at many points along the way) feel like you're never going to make it.

Then one day you will. Slowly things will start to change. The pain will feel a little less jagged and unbearable, and you will find a way to make meaning of your loss that has previously felt completely unfair and meaningless. Of course, you may never find a 'good' explanation for why you lost your baby, but eventually your soul will be able to understand that all of this happened for a reason. *Whatever you decide that to be.*

One of the surprising things I found about grief is how we need others to get through it. We need their stories to mirror back to us our own thoughts and our feelings. They help us understand our own grief.

If we try to battle grief alone we get so lost in the fog of it that we can't see who we are now, or who we'll eventually be on the other side. It can feel like a lonely road that we are destined to walk on forever. It can be difficult to understand our own feelings and it can feel like no one else understands us either.

But when we feel heard and understood, we can start to make sense of what has happened. I can't explain how it works. But being seen and understood by others helps us to find a way to make the absolute awfulness of our situation feel somewhat okay.

Truthfully, this is a horrible shitty club to be a part of. This I-lost-a-baby-and-life-feels-fucking-unfair-club. But one day you *will* find your way to the other side of it. You never get to leave the club, of course. But you'll know that you're starting to get there when you find yourself welcoming others to it. Offering others who go through this loss your story and your love, as I hope this book will do for you.

Before we get into my story, I just want to put it out there that at the time of writing these words I do not know whether or not there will be a baby at the end of this book. And that's really not the point. I have not written this book because I know the secrets to overcoming all of the barriers to infertility and how to get your baby. I'm sorry if that's what you came here for. *That is not this book.* As I write these words today I am unsure whether I'll ever hold another newborn child of my own in my arms. But I'm determined to find a way back to happy anyway.

The aim of this book is to hopefully share how we can go on living and loving, regardless of whether our story includes a baby or not. It's about whether we can open ourselves back up to the joy of life and all of it's brutal and amazing experiences, knowing that there are no guarantees that it will all turn out okay. And maybe it will also be about being brave enough to open ourselves up to love again, when we know that loss may be the outcome.

I think we all want to believe that we will get our happy ending, *but what if we don't?* At what point do we need to make the decision to find our happiness regardless of the outcome? *And can it be done?*

This book is not about overcoming the grief of losing a baby. It's about finding a way to go on living a full life anyway. It's about finding a way to make peace with your losses. It's about doing the work to heal your heart and creating a life that makes you happy not despite your losses, *but because of them.*

How to read this book

Of course there is no right or wrong way to read a book. Read it from start to finish. Or dip in and out as the mood strikes you. In the early days I often found that I couldn't read for too long on this topic or else my mood would become too dark. Then at times when I felt alone and incredibly sad, being able to pick up books by authors who clearly understood how I felt helped to soothe the pain a little.

You'll notice that this book is written in four parts.

Part One shares my personal story. I've attempted to write as honestly and openly as I can about my experience and feelings after losing our babies. This part was written over a couple of years. It starts not long after the loss of our second baby and spans almost two years of our journey. Many of the words in this section come straight from my journal.

I share my reflections and feelings from within the raw pain of loss, and of the days, months and even years that follow. While there has been some editing to make it legible, I have tried not to edit how I felt in the moment so that perhaps you can find a little of yourself in my words.

In **Part Two** you will find stories from women in my community. Strong, brave, incredible women who reached out to me in my darkest moments to lend their light when I had none. In this section I share their stories of hope and survival.

In **Part Three** you'll find my advice on some of the trickier parts of living after losing a baby. I've tried to speak to areas I struggled with the most and looked for information on in the early days. I hope that you can approach this section like advice from a friend. Take it or leave it. Use what resonates and leave the rest.

Part Four is a mini-course of words and practices to help you through the first 40 days.

Journalling and self-reflection has been an incredibly important part of my healing. I started writing every morning before I would start my day. It really helped to give me the space to work through my grief. Writing helped to get 'the madness' out of my head and heart, before my days of having to *get on with it* started.

These prompts will help you to connect with yourself and your grief every day. This can be confronting at first. But I've found that you either give grief the attention it wants or it will pop up elsewhere in your life and *demand it*.

PART 1 - MY STORY

9th December 2016

It's been a week since we lost our second baby. A baby whose gender we'll never know. Whose hands we'll never hold and whose name still remains a mystery to me. How do I name someone who was here for such a short time? What name do you give someone who will never hear it called and who will never write it proudly on his artwork to stick on the fridge?

We named the first boy we lost, Orion, for the constellation. I wanted to look up to the sky and see him there. I'd already picked the name before I knew it's meaning. A Google search from my bed in the early hours one morning told me it meant "rising in the sky, dawning". These are exactly the words Andrew used to explain what had happened to our four year old at the time, so it felt fitting.

Naming Orion though felt very different. I was 16 weeks along. I gave birth to him and held him in my hands. In the darkened hospital room, I touched his tiny fingers and stared at his tiny face while tears streamed down mine. This time, the only time I saw my baby was through the blurry black and white image of the ultrasound. By then his heart had already stopped. His soul had already left.

This time I chose to have a D&C. I couldn't face waiting up to 12 weeks for my body to realise it was no longer making a viable (goddam I hate that word) baby and release him naturally. Nor could I bear inserting the medication again to make my body expel his tiny body. I couldn't go through another birth experience like Orion's.

Especially not with the memory of last time so fresh in my mind. The horror of it all. I wish I could sugar-coat it in some way for you, but I really only have negative memories of that night. In the thick of it I remember thinking *Why did I ever explain Eamon's birth as traumatic - nothing can compare to this horror of birthing a baby that you so desperately want, but cannot have. Nothing can compare to the horror of a birth and death, all at the same time."*

I remember flashing hot and cold and passing out from it all. I have memories of my life flashing before my eyes and I felt like I was dying. Perhaps a tad overdramatic looking back, but in the moment, I felt like it would be my last. I felt like I couldn't bear life anymore. I couldn't deal with the physical or emotional pain in that moment.

I guess that's why I passed out. It was my body's way of finding momentary relief. I felt like I wasn't strong enough to survive this loss. I wanted to give up. For that moment the pain in my heart and the emptiness of my belly ceased to exist. I was nothing and nowhere and yet I remember feeling peaceful.

I woke up on the bed. They gave me a shot of something in my leg and I cried out in pain, but really I didn't care. I just wanted to sleep. They were taking me to theatre because the placenta hadn't come out and my cervix had already shut. I remember feeling so angry. I had just gone through *all of that* only to have to go into theatre anyway?!

The rest of the day is mostly a blur. Except for a few moments that stand out so clearly in my mind.

1. The theatre nurse congratulating me on the birth of my baby and asking me what I'd had. (He had read 'placenta removal' on my chart and not looked closely enough at the details.)

2. The looks on the faces of the other nurses as they tried to tell that nurse what he had just said to a woman whose baby was dead.

3. The kindness of the post-op nurses who worked really hard to make me smile.

4. Leaving the maternity ward empty handed as babies cried out in rooms around me.

Even though it was only 7 months ago, I can't actually remember how I got through those first few days and weeks after we came home from losing Orion. I guess it must have been just one moment at a time, as I feel like I'm doing again now.

This time it feels harder.

Now I have the added bonus of all the questions that are running through my head.

What if you lose the next baby too?
What if you can never have another?
Maybe you're only meant to have two?
What if you can't even get pregnant again?
What if Andrew doesn't want to go through it all again?
Shouldn't you just be grateful for the two healthy boys you already have?
Maybe your body needs a break for a while?
What if you take a break and try again in 3 years and still it happens again anyway?

And on and on and around it goes. Like some sort of horror-merry-go-round that I can't get off.

14th December 2016

It's been two weeks. Two weeks since that moment where I lay on the ultrasound chair hoping for good news, only to have them quickly squashed with the words *'It doesn't look good.'*

I'm not coping well today. Although I'm not 100% sure that I even know what 'coping well' looks like anymore. I feel snappy and frustrated with my boys. Rory, my 1 year old, is going through a particularly delightful stage of crying about everything. Crying because he doesn't want to go in the car. Crying because he doesn't want to get out of the car. Crying because he doesn't want me. Crying because he does want me.

I feel like a total hypocrite crying for a baby I never knew, while feeling frustrated at the one right in front of me. Like somehow this is all a test, because I am not doing a good enough job at home. I know it's not, but in my darkest moments this is how it feels.

I'm not proud of how I'm mothering at the minute. I find myself desperately seeking distraction to numb myself from the grief. This means I'm also struggling to be here in this moment, which is the only place my children know how to operate.

I'm writing this now after sending the boys down to 'help' Andrew in the garage. I've reached my limit for today and need a break. I can hear them from hear fighting and squabbling over things they probably shouldn't even be touching.

I'd love to be able to tell you how these losses have shown me how precious my boys are and how they have completely changed me as a mother. In some ways, and at some times, this is true. Right now though, *today*, it's not. I want to be honest about this part too.

Right now I feel like I want to curl inside a shell all by myself. I want to retreat from the world and pretend like I never even had plans for next year *when the baby comes.*

30th December 2016

Keeping a relationship strong is hard at the best of times. Navigating a relationship after losing a baby is epically hard. Doing so when you feel like you are crumbling and there are no answers to anything feels hopeless.

He grieves differently. As much as I want to be supportive of how he needs to grieve sometimes I doubt that he is feeling anything at all.

Sometimes I want to shout at him - *But aren't you dying inside? Where is your sadness? Where are your tears?!'*

In these moments I doubt the depth of his feelings for our baby in comparison to mine.

This feels like a shitty thing to say *(or write)* out loud. But there it is.

I feel like this hasn't hurt him as much as it's hurt me. This makes me feel incredibly selfish and alone.

You would expect a shared loss like this would pull a couple together. I know of friends who have been on the IVF train together and they have rallied against the challenges they needed to tackle *together.*

But for the most part it isn't like that for us. He carries on. Working. Building stuff for our house (which I am beginning to suspect is his method of 'coping' as he's started new projects days after both losses). Doing all of his regular things. While I feel like I crumble into myself. I cry. I don't eat. I just want to stop thinking, to stop remembering, to stop feeling so empty.

Some days, I do feel a connection with him over our losses. In those rare moments when he cracks open a little and shares what is on his heart. These moments usually come after I break and share my latest lack of coping and how his indifference feels like he doesn't care.

In those moments he gives me something. But it feels like I have to draw it out of him and I really don't have the strength for that.

He told me recently how he feels like after what we've been through nothing can pull us apart. I remember thinking at the time… *'Really?! I feel like we're already crumbling.'*

I feel like I am the only one still hurting. He goes on with his days and never cracks. I crumble and break regularly. A burnt piece of toast can set me off for the whole day.

I am trying to talk more. To say *"I'm sad."* in an effort to explain some of my more depressive behaviours.

He often responds with *"About what?"*.

To which I want to scream *"How can you ask that question? Isn't it obvious? Aren't you sad too? Aren't your insides churning from the sadness of it all?"*

Or am I all alone? Just like I suspected?

6th January 2017

I'm beginning to feel frustrated that my body hasn't started cycling again yet. After losing Orion I felt pregnant for most of the year. It was like my body didn't get the message and continued to pretend I was still carrying a baby. My boobs hurt. I still carried the extra weight. But at least my body started cycling as normal almost immediately.

This time, my body got the message straight away that I was no longer pregnant. My boobs disappeared the very next day and the weight fell off me. But still no cycle. We're almost up to six weeks.

I feel like I have permanent PMS. I'm cranky. I'm picking holes in my relationship that don't exist. I want to snap every time someone asks if I'm okay. I want to shout *'NO I'M NOT BLOODY OKAY!'*

But I am. Or at least I know I will be.

It's just this swirling tide of emotions in my belly sometimes makes me feel overwhelmed by it all. Like it's bigger than me and I will never be able to get off this horror show of a ride.

14th January 2017

I've been blaming myself. Not outwardly. My head knows that there wasn't anything I could have done. My heart isn't quite convinced though. Late at night when the house is quiet I often feel a rush of guilt. I look at my body in disgust for not being able to keep my babies safe.

My counsellor called me on it the other day. *'You feel guilty, as if your body failed you.'* she said matter-of-factly, as if she already knew.

What followed was a conversation about all of those ugly thoughts that I'd been hiding. I aired out the stench of them with her.

"My body did this."
"How can I ever trust it again?"
"What is wrong with me?"
"I am a failure?"

In doing so they became a little less scary. A little less truthful. I no longer felt like I had to wholeheartedly believe them. Though I have to admit they are still definitely lurking there.

It certainly hasn't been an immediate forgivingness of my body. That is something I'm still working on. But admitting that I felt insanely guilty about it all, felt like a positive first step.

18th January 2017

I did not grow up with a religion, but I would describe myself as spiritual. I believe we are souls having a human experience. I believe that after we pass away, there is something else for us.

I don't know what that is.

I don't know if it is reincarnation. I don't know whether I believe in the idea of heaven.

I do know that I believe that we are here to learn.

I heard this idea the other day that our souls come together each lifetime to learn the next step in their evolution.

Someone said that maybe these souls, our babies, only need those first few stages of development at this time in their journey. Or maybe they came for such a short time because our soul had lessons to learn? Whatever they may be.

I like the sound of this but it still makes me unbelievably sad.

I don't know if I believe this.

But I do believe that our babies, if and when we get to meet them again, would not want us to stop living simply because their time had come to an end. And if I do get to meet them somewhere, in another life, or maybe this one. I want to live in a way that makes them proud.

30th January 2017

So... here we go again.

I'm shocked to be here so quickly. In all honestly we weren't actually 'trying' for another baby. Though obviously, we also weren't trying to *not* have a baby either.

I hesitated over whether I should share this news. Last time I wanted to keep it completely hush hush, despite having only recently told everyone how bullshit I think the 12 week wait is. I remember feeling that in some way I would 'jinx it' by announcing too soon.

But the not telling is just as unhelpful.

Either way, telling or not telling, losing a baby is a hopelessly tragic situation. People either know and you have to explain what happened. Or they don't know and you have to explain why you're no longer 'yourself' and why you're so sad all the time.

Or you don't tell and explain anything and you feel detached and alone in your grief.

So pretty much, it's a lose, lose, lose situation.

So this time, I'm just going to be present with the whole truth of it and see how that plays out.

So here we are. I am pregnant again. Barely, *just*. 5 weeks by my *guesstimate*. A third pregnancy in just under a year. My fifth pregnancy altogether.

My body knows how to do this well now. I already feel uncomfortable with my yoga tights pressing into my belly. I feel like I'm already showing. Although after our second loss late last year, I lost a fair bit of weight so there really is no where else for it to go now.

I'm equal parts terrified and hesitantly optimistic.

I'm also exhausted down to my bones.

I've gone back to *my* GP this time. The one who I saw throughout Rory's pregnancy, but who I avoided after losing Orion. I can't explain why I didn't go back to her before. It certainly wasn't my greatest idea to instead go to a random doctor who didn't have English as a first language. I remember trying to explain to him I was pregnant but *'Please don't say that word as I have two kids here with me. One who knows that word well, and I'm trying to protect him this time.'*

Perhaps I just had a bit of a mental block around her because she delivered the bad news that first time. Or the start of it anyway. I think maybe I just didn't want to deal with the loss at all last time. Like if I pretended I'd never lost a baby then I didn't have to deal with the sadness and I could just pretend that this next pregnancy was a completely normal happy one.

Obviously the 'avoid strategy' didn't work. So this time I'm just facing it all head on. I went back to her this week and I had a big cry as she said all of the right things. 'Hesitantly positive' are her words. She decided they will be our mantra and I like that right from the start she has included herself in this process. I realise that I was really missing that support last time.

Last time I showed up to a random GP to get the confirmation and referrals.

I then went to another random OB (one who did the scan during our pregnancy for Orion but that I'd only met once) only to be given more bad news that there was no heartbeat at 10 weeks.

I was then sent to the hospital to meet a random midwife who talked us through deciding on taking medication to bring on labour, waiting for a natural miscarriage or D&C.

We chose to have a D&C which was performed by another doctor who I'd never met before and hope to never meet again.

I had about half an hour of support in hospital recovery by more random nurses before being sent home with the recommendation that I go back and see *my GP* in the next couple of weeks.

Looking back I can see it really was the wrong decision to not have people on my side.

This still feels HUGE and scary, but I'm pleased that I'm not facing it alone this time.

3rd February 2017

Rory has been the light of my days recently. It's been a pretty dark week. The other night I sleep-walked for the first time in years. I woke wandering the house in tears looking for my babies. Needless to say there wasn't much sleep after that.

I feel like I'm not sure my heart can handle any more sadness. (And no universe this is NOT a *'Go on try me'* statement this is a *'I'm done'* announcement.

Upswing only from now on thank-you-very-much.

6th February 2017

Sunrise feels different when everything is falling apart.

I woke up to what feels like the start of my period this morning. I'm not sure where to even go from here?

Every other time I've found out there was something wrong was at during an ultrasound.

I'm praying my baby is okay. Or at least for the strength to survive another loss.

7th February 2017

If you're trying to get pregnant or are currently pregnant, whether happily or nervously, it's time to step away from the internet.

The problem with turning to google for advice on anything is that it will inevitably turn up the answer you are looking for.

I know, I know. Sounds excellent. Exactly what you wanted, right?

Unfortunately, no. It doesn't find the answer to your question. It finds the answer you want to hear.

Google is the too scared to tell you the hard truth friend that you turn to when you're feeling doubtful and want to be pandered to.

I know this because every time I've turned to Google when I've had issues with pregnancies over the last year, he told me everything I wanted to hear.

The statistics said my chances of bad news were low so it's going to be okay. *Google didn't prepare me for the fact that someone had to be the statistic.*

Google told me there are thousands of women who've had the same thing happen to them and everything was okay. Google forgot to show me the results with all the other women who've had the same thing and it didn't turn out fine.

Whatever your experience, there is someone out there who has had the exact same thing happen and it has turned out well. Or it hasn't.

Interestingly, it's only when things haven't gone well for me and I've started looking for the other side of the story that my searches have showed up that option as well.

So now I'm less trusting of Google. I'm better at searching for both sides of the coin and ultimately I can find every answer imaginable and therefore none at all.

So here we are again. I had some spotting over the weekend. I tried to stay calm and tell myself this happened in Eamon's pregnancy too and he is more than fine. Monday morning though I woke to more of a gush (but in hindsight still not actually that much).

I got in to see my Obstetrician for a scan yesterday morning. I fully anticipated to be told the baby had already passed. (It seems I'm now squarely in the camp of err on the side of the negative now in order to not have my hopes completely obliterated by bad news. Sad but true.)

But there on the screen was a perfectly beating little heart inside a perfect little bean.

Relief. Disbelief.

We came home and had lunch. The sick feeling in my stomach that had been there all weekend was finally gone. Andrew left for work.

The bleeding worsened. It was just myself and Rory home. He is obsessed with the toilet at the moment because we have just started toilet training. He screamed outside the door as I sat and felt like it was all over. I passed some very large clots but I was only in there for a few minutes.

I changed my pad and went outside to cry with Rory, ring my Mum and Andrew, and lie down. The bleeding was like a heavy period for a few hours then slowed and this morning is back to only light spotting.

I'm at a complete loss. Is that it? Is it over?

Is the baby gone? Surely it couldn't have happened so quickly?

Google tells me with 100% certainty that my baby could be gone, no pain and the fastest miscarriage in history. It also tells me with certainty that I could go in to have another scan and we see the heartbeat of our baby, blissfully unaware of all the drama.

Yes it's definitely time for me to step away from looking to the internet for answers. I'm also at a loss for where to look for actual answers. My GP only works Wednesday and Friday and is impossible to get into. I can't get a hold of my OB and even if I did, do I even want another scan? Perhaps that's what stirred things up in the first place?

I'm unsure what I should be doing? Bed rest? Getting on with life and just seeing what happens? I feel like I can't teach yoga because what if it worsens mid-class? In all honesty, yoga is the last thing I feel like doing. I guess it's back to the couch?

I'm stuck in the in-between. The wait and see. The put everything on hold and wait place. It feels like the worst place to be.

It feels like life is on hold. I over-analyse and agonise over every symptom, every twinge. I go to the toilet every five minutes to wipe and check for blood. Are my boobs sorer or softer than yesterday?

The in-between consumes my every thought. It's hard to make plans. It's hard to think beyond the next minute, let alone make plans for coming weeks or months.

I've been in this in-between before. When I was pregnant with Orion and we were waiting for test results. Then to be told the bad news that he was not going to be the healthy happy baby we'd imagined and it was up to us to make the decision to go full term or deliver early. It felt like a cruel joke that the world was playing on us, to make us decide to terminate a much-wanted baby. I spent a lot of time bawling and asking to no one in particular *Why is this happening to us?' 'What did we do to deserve this?'*

Now I am in the in-between again. Some bleeding, followed by a positive scan. Followed by more serious bleeding. Everyone is telling me to keep hope. But I feel like I need to protect my heart. I feel like it needs the protection of my doubt, of my already assuming the worst, so that the worst might hurt a little less.

9th February 2017

I went for another ultrasound today. Baby was completely oblivious to all the drama. We saw our healthy little jellybean, heart beating away perfectly.

Seriously *what a week*. It feels like I've run a marathon, but all I've done is sat and slept.

Only 33 more weeks to go!

11th February 2017

My first two pregnancies can only be described as nothing short of ideal. (If only I'd known how great I had it then so I could have appreciated it more).

I was very healthy.

I only had minor morning sickness.

I was 100% confident in my ability to grow a healthy baby.

The only discomfort I had was some pelvic pain with Rory from about 20 weeks.

I practiced strong yoga right 'til the end of both pregnancies with no problem.

This one, after last week, and of course with the experience of the last two, is a whole other ball-game.

I've never felt so disconnected from my body and so lacking in trust of its ability to grow a healthy baby.

I feel like I am waiting for bad news, for confirmation.

I visit the toilet 100 times per day to check to see whether the bleeding is worse or has it finally stopped?

I'm fearful of going too far from home in case the bleeding gets heavier again.

I'm afraid to move too much in fear of making anything worse.

My belly is tender and swollen.

Some days I feel incredibly sick all day long and feel mildly calmed by this sign of a healthy pregnancy. My nausea makes me want to lie horizontal, eat all the food and not move too much. Then the next day all sickness vanishes and I am left anxiously looking for any sign of it. At the same time also wanting to lie horizontal to avoid over stressing my already stressed body and stress-eating all the food. (Good times).

For someone whose work involves teaching other women to trust their body during pregnancy, this is a particularly difficult experience. Though obviously something I needed to learn. (But seriously universe, I've had enough with the lessons now thank-you-very-much.)

My body already feels sore and stiff from so little movement in the last week. I feel tired in my bones. Both from all the stress, the first trimester and also that sloth-like feeling that comes from lack of movement.

I have that first trimester daze where I can't seem to focus on any one thing, nor make conversation because I feel like my brain is constantly elsewhere. Constantly worrying about other things.

I wish I could tell you I had the secret to learning how to trust your body again after you've lost babies. But I don't have any of these answers. Not right now anyway.

I'm trusting that it's okay to be here, in the not knowing. Maybe I will find the answers along the way? Or maybe I won't. The only thing I know for sure, is that I will get to the other side. That this experience won't be forever. That one day all this anxiety and stress and worry will fade and that maybe I will struggle to remember what all the fuss was about.

26th February 2017

Life feels endlessly on hold.

10 weeks today. This is as far as we made it with our last baby so I guess I should feel positive about that.

Although even now that little voice in the back of my mind says *'But you didn't really make it that far. You just didn't know until then. This could be the same.'*

I do feel different this time.

I feel nauseous all the time. I feel very pregnant in my belly and in my boobs. Definitely more than last time anyway.

I can't ever remember analysing all the symptoms more than I have during this pregnancy. Some days I feel like I'm driving myself completely crazy.

6th March 2017

I have an Obstetrician appointment in half and hour.

I am terrified.
In some ways I feel like I'd rather stay in the unknowing.

Please let our baby be perfectly healthy.

Please let our baby be perfectly healthy.
Please let our baby be perfectly healthy.

7th March 2017

It's another dark day.

You would think the sharp shock of it would be less by now.

It's not.

It's just as raw and as painful third time round.
I think the darkness that follows is a little scarier now though.

First time around I felt like there was still hope, still another chance - we just had to try again.

Now I don't even believe in my own strength to open myself up again to that risk.

I feel so lost.

How can this be happening again?
Didn't I do everything I could?
I literally surrendered everything.
What more am I meant to do?

8th March 2017

I've been awake since 4am. The exhaustion from yesterday ran out and now I have to deal with the eleven billion thoughts rattling round my head.

The most beautiful sunrise just appeared in the sky for a short five minutes. And with it this thought - *"There will always be a new dawn and all the beauty that comes with it. But before the dawn there will always be the dark."*

So today I will hug my boys before I go into the hospital for yet another D & C. I'll be there when they get home from school and kindy.

A little sore, a little tender, but also achingly grateful.

For all of it.

9th March 2017

I feel like I should write something profound about International Women's day but in all honesty I can barely form a coherent thought at the moment, other than an angry stream of thoughts at the universe in general.

I have no big statement to make about how women are changing the world. But I can tell you how they're changing mine.

This week the women in my life have loved my boys like their own while I've slept.

They've held my hand as I cried.

Women I've never met have cared for me in the darkness of a hospital room.

They've left dinner on my doorstep.

They've named a star for my babies and filled my house with flowers.

Women have sent me messages just to say they didn't have any words to say.

They've kept me in their thoughts and prayers.

It is in the smallest of acts that I feel the most loved.

Women are stronger than we even know.

10th March 2017

How did we even get here? I feel a bit confused.

Last I remember I was enjoying having two boys. I had everything I'd ever wanted. A beautiful family. A house by the beach. Work I enjoyed. Enough money to do the fun things we wanted to do. Support around me. Good friends.

I can't even remember deciding that a third child was a good idea for us. The before and after of that moment in time now blur together. What made me come to that conclusion? What brought me to the point that decided our family wasn't complete without a third?

Now it feels like we're in too far.

I feel like I've spent the entire last year thinking about a third baby. It makes me sad because it now feels like time wasted. Time that I should have spent focused on the two beautiful boys in front of me. They have certainly been by my side and front of mind but I feel like in some ways I've robbed myself of the enjoyment of that. I haven't felt complete within our little family because I've been so focused on trying to have our third.

I have one distinct memory of total contentment before we lost Orion. I was putting Rory to bed (which consisted of lying next to him pretending to sleep while he did gymnastics on the bed beside me). I remember this overwhelming feeling of gratitude for the family we had created. I had our sleepy babe within me, Eamon who was reading with Andrew in the other room and our crazy blondie practicing his somersaults. Everything felt perfect. As if it were meant to be.

I'm now at a point I don't recognise. How is it possible I've been through three losses? How is it possible that I have more babies lost to me than in my arms? How did I arrive here?

Of course, I remember the journey. It is burned in my heart and body.

I have constant flashbacks of various moments when I haven't managed to fill every single moment with busy-ness.

An obstetrician saying to me after having repairs for a third degree tear after Rory's birth – *"Don't worry this doesn't mean you won't be able to have any more children."* I remember feeling confused at the time. That thought had never once occurred to me, so I wondered why he was even addressing it. It now stands out as something significant in time.

An energy worker I visited after losing Orion who said to me *"He says, when you're ready, he'll send the others."* I now wish I'd clarified - *'Will there be any more living children?'*

At what point is it time to make the decision to get off this road? At what point do you put it all aside and say *'Enough!'*

What I have is enough. We are enough. Just our little bunch. At what point do you know this is the right decision for you and not just one made out of fear of continuing to try…and failing. At what point is it time to quit while you're ahead, or not?

In many ways, we could still be just scraping the surface of this journey. We've had no fertility testing. I've only had basic testing to see what the problem could be (and they found nothing). This potentially could be a very long road if we continue to go down it.

Is this a road we even want to be on? How did we even get here?

14th March 2017

So here we are, with three little stars in the sky.

It seems unimaginably horrible and cruel and yet I know (now) I am not unique in this experience. After losing one baby many women reached out and told me of their losses. Some mentioned numbers then, most simply gave me words to let me know I was not alone.

Now that I've lost multiple babies, I have become a part of a brand new shitty club. Perhaps they were protecting me before. Knowing that I needed to focus on the positive, not on the likelihood that I could experience this pain many times over before I would get to hold my baby. I'm not sure whether to thank them for that, *or not*.

Mostly I find myself feeling very lost right now. I spent most of yesterday starting and stopping random jobs around the house. I couldn't really focus or motivate myself to do anything. I'm restless. Seeking distraction in all the usual places, but nothing seems to take the edge off anymore.

A wise woman wrote to me the other day to say *'You need to water the flowers, not the weeds'.*

At first I thought, *'Isn't that what I've been doing?'* Haven't I been trying to make a positive out of this whole shitty experience? I've been trying to share my heart. Not only because it feels helpful to share the thoughts that rattle around my head so that I don't feel so crazy and alone, but also because I know it helps others too.

But perhaps, in a way, this is also watering the weeds? I've been focusing on the negative, the sadness of it all.

Haven't I?

I've mostly been sharing how scared and anxious I was in pregnancy. It wasn't a story of hope. Yes, I stand by the fact that this is the honest truth of my story, and I don't want to be sharing a fake glossy version of anything. But by focusing on this, by sharing how scared and anxious I was – did I make the weeds grow?

I remember reading comments on some of my blog posts over the last month and thinking *'How can you be so positive?'* or *'How can you be so optimistic after everything?'* Wishing I could feel just a touch of it myself.

I think my friends, there lies a problem.

I've lost my optimism. I've lost my ability to see the possibility in anything. Even non-baby related things, I find myself finding all the negatives before I even think of the positives.

I've lost hope. Along with it, I've lost those feelings of love and excitement for life in general.

Do you remember what it feels like to feel excited over something as simple as the crisp morning air reminding you that it's nearly Easter?

I don't.

I feel like I've been holding my breath. Like I wasn't allowing myself to feel anything, trying to protect myself from being hurt again. And look how well that turned out.

Do you remember what it feels like to plan life around holidays and things you want to do, rather than around pregnancies and due dates.

I don't.

For too long now, my head has been quietly calculating how many weeks I'll be, or due dates, or dates I know that I'll be too upset to do anything.

Do you remember what it feels like to just do things for you?

I don't.

All of my self-care over the past month, has been because I was trying to take care of this baby. None of it was for me.

Now that I've lost another, I find myself struggling to even care. I find myself asking – '*Why should I bother?*' My head knows why, but my heart is too sad to listen at the minute.

I've decided it's time to take a break. 6 months. 12 months. Perhaps indefinitely. I'm not really sure yet.

Even just writing those words hurts my heart. It feels like giving up. It feels like giving in to the possibility that maybe there will never be a third baby for us. Perhaps that's a reality I need to face though. Or maybe just a reality I need to at least accept, in order to find my hope and optimism for life again.

I feel like I need to get back to living, rather than waiting. I need to remember what it feels like to be blissfully happy without the added extra of *When we have this baby'* lurking in the back of my mind. Or even *When we fall pregnant'* for that matter.

I want to make lists of things I want to do that aren't determined by whether I'm pregnant or not, or whether I have a new babyor not.

I want to remember how to feel grateful for what I already have. My head knows it, but my heart is struggling to feel.

16th March 2017

It's possible I have a drinking problem? Not the 'drink all day' version. But I've noticed I'm starting to rely on having a couple of glasses of wine each night to take the edge off the pain and help me sleep.

If I'm not completely exhausted and a little bit tipsy by the time my head hits the pillow, I lie awake and cry for hours. Is it a problem if I'm aware of what I'm doing or only if I'm doing it unconsciously?

I really must try to not have anything to drink tomorrow night and find another way to numb out before bed. Meditation. A couple of extra episodes of something on Netflix. Reading 'til my eyes fall asleep. Anything other than wine really.

17th March 2017

Failed at my own resolution and had a glass of red wine last night (or two or three). Will try again tomorrow.

18th March 2017

This being human business is messy, isn't it? In my next life I'm coming back as something peaceful and uncomplicated. Like a sunset. Or a star. Hell, I'd even take a rock at this point if it were peaceful.

19th March 2017

Going out at the moment feels like too much effort. Sleep evades me. Even writing and yoga feel too damn hard.

But books and other people's drama, that keeps my mind busy in a good way, which is exactly what I need right now. At least for the next hour while Rory sleeps anyway.

And then, thank god for climb-the-wall two year olds who will keep me so busy I can't remember.

20th March 2017

Andrew and I have reached a new level of broken. The last week has shown us exactly how far apart our completely different paths of grief have taken us. I'm not proud to admit. In fact, if you'd asked me a couple of weeks ago how we were going I would have said pretty well, *all things considered.*

But this week we both cracked and broke. It was probably well overdue, but that doesn't mean it hurts any less. I've been telling him for a while now how alone I've felt in so much of this. But until today I don't feel like he has really understood what I meant by that.

Whenever I've said that he would say *'But I am here. I've been by your side through all of it, you're not alone.'* I guess what I've been meaning was that I felt emotionally alone. He has been present physically, but emotionally elsewhere.

Not that I can really blame him. I've been doing a lot of this myself. Seeking distraction and comfort from everywhere else but him. We didn't really even talk about our last two babies.

We fell pregnant and then both held our breaths.

When it all came tumbling down, I broke and he held it together.

He believed that was his role - to hold it all together for us. To me, that felt like he didn't care. It felt like none of this really affected him at all because his life literally went on just as it always had the very next day.

Whereas each time I've felt the paralysis of grief more and more. I've wanted to retreat from the world. Conversation feels too hard and not worth the effort. Yet he goes straight back to the gym. To going to see a footy game. To organising social things. As if nothing has happened.

This weekend I think he has finally been able to see that holding it together for me has actually made things between us worse. He tells me he has broken down many times. At work. In the car. By himself. But because I haven't seen any of it I've felt completely alone in my grief.

I feel like we've hit our rock bottom. Though maybe it's a bottom we needed to hit. Now that we're here, the only way out is to hold each other's hands and help each other up.

22nd March 2017

I tried to go shopping today for a dress to wear to a wedding this weekend. Normally I would just wear something from my wardrobe but my body is still in-between and none of my regular clothes really fit at the moment. My body hasn't quite realised yet that I'm not pregnant.

My belly is still soft and round. My boobs still full. My legs and arms are still holding onto the extra weight that was supposed to be feeding my baby.

I spent three hours at the shops, wandering in and out, trying on clothes and getting more and more worked up. By the end I was ready to burst into tears and did exactly that when I made it back to the safety of my car.

It feels bad enough that I have to feel the sadness of losing a baby, but to also have to deal with the physical reminders as well is just cruel. I struggle to not feel disgust when I look in the mirror. What only a few weeks ago brought me so much joy, my growing belly, a general thickening, is now just another painful reminder of what I am not.

I'd love to not even go to this wedding, but I don't think that would go down well with Andrew. We need the night out together. We need to do something fun and light. Though I already know I will spend most of the night plastering on a happy face while pushing down thoughts that make me want to cry.

My brain had already calculated the number of weeks I would be by this date. As it had done for every other special occasion we had written on the calendar this year.

27th March 2017

I started packing up baby things today. I ugly cried through the whole process. I feel like I just want the reminders out of my sight. I don't want to walk past the spare cupboard and see all the boxes of baby things. I don't want to be reminded of the fact that we are meant to be using them right now, but aren't. I don't want to have to reach past the cot to get the vacuum cleaner and then bawl while cleaning the floors.

I'm done. It feels like a strange form of self-torture, but for some reason I feel compelled to clear it all out.

Andrew says I shouldn't. He says to leave it because we will try again later in the year. He knows how much I want a third.

But I guess I'm now questioning, why?

I definitely know that if I said I was done after two, he would have been happily done.

Hell, even if I'd said I was done after one, he would of been like 'Ok, great. *Let's move with the next phase of our life'*.

If I'm only doing this for me, yet it's causing me so much pain - is it worth it?

28th March 2017

I asked Eamon to unpack the dishwasher this morning. I'd been crying but I thought I'd pulled myself together well enough that he wouldn't notice.

He came over and said *'Okay, but first I think I need to give you a hug'*.

I often wonder how this whole experience will shape him as a man.

Maybe this is one small gift in this whole shitty experience?

29th March 2017

This entry includes questions and answers I wrote to myself in my journal at the time. I started writing my morning pages by asking questions and answering them with whatever flowed out of my head and onto the page.

I tried not to think and analyse it. Maybe try to do the same as you read this now (not over-analyse). Otherwise you'll probably think I'm a total nut job. I include this here now because I think it speaks to the fact that even in our darkest moments we already hold all the wisdom on healing that we need.

How do I get out of this hole?

Focus on you. Make yourself happy.

But how? I don't know what makes me happy anymore?

Stop fighting. Follow what feels good. Speak up when you're not okay. Love. Forgive. Try again.

What about my work? It's so painful now. Do I let that go? Forget about it? Do something else?

Does it make you happy?

I don't know anymore.

I think you do. It's just hidden under the hurt. It's hiding behind your lack of confidence, your insecurity. Nothing feels predictable or safe anymore. But that's reality.

If the worst can happen, so can the best. You've got to find a way to believe that again. Believe that you deserve the best as well as the worst. You deserve to feel the way you want to feel. Don't stop or accept anything less.

30th March 2017

This last week or so I've been laying pretty low. I'm still not physically 100% and although I am back teaching yoga, I mostly only leave the house for that and school drop off. I feel like each time I've lost a baby I end up with a small case of social anxiety. I want to avoid all people and social situations because it's just too painful and awkward.

At school drop off the other day one of the Mums asked *'How are you? Tired?'*.

I just answered, *'Yes pretty tired'* and thought how strange that wording was to ask an almost stranger.

It wasn't until we were leaving that I remembered that I'd met her at a birthday party a couple of weeks ago and had told her I was pregnant. Now I've missed that awkward opening to tell her I lost the baby. I hope that I don't see her again anytime soon and she just works it out with time. See, painful and awkward.

1st April 2017

It feels completely self-indulgent to write a list of things that I want to do just to make me happy. But I've found that if I don't have an actual focus or goal, I just wander the house aimlessly, or lie on the couch feeling lost and sad.

So I decided I needed a list to tick off. Something to give me some direction and purpose to my days. So here it is. My 'happy list.' A list of 20 things to do that are just for me. 20 things that have no purpose other than to help me feel happy again.

1   Take a solo retreat.
2   Try aerial yoga.
3   Get a massage.
4   Take a kid-free weekend away with Andrew.
5   Make the ensuite renovation happen.
6   Take a family holiday away and completely switch off.
7   Continue reading a book per week.
8   Eat veggies from our own veggie patch.
9   Take myself out on weekly coffee & book writing dates.
10 Feel strong and healthy in my body again.
11 Full moon sunset drinks on the beach.
12 Organise a ladies nights out.
13 Try Barre Body.
14 Take an online course in something... Just. For. Me.
15 Pick up my real camera again regularly instead of just my iPhone.
16 Date nights x 2.
17 Go to the movies.
18 Bonfire on the beach.
19 Fix up / decorate the front verandah.
20 Redo our bedroom with new linen/ clear it out.

3rd April 2017

The sun is finally shining today (although I'm not sure for how long) and Rory actually woke up happy, rather than his usual rolling around on the floor and whinging. Maybe it's going to be a good day.

So these morning pages I've been doing. I've been able to write page upon page about our crumbling marriage. How difficult I'm finding motherhood. Detailed descriptions about every other problem in my life.

Yet I can't seem to write a word of my book.*

Or perhaps the question is - *do I even want to anymore?* At the start of the year it felt so important. Like it would somehow right the wrong of losing another baby. But then I lost again and realised nothing will do that. Not ever. ***It will always be wrong.***

My babies will always be dead. No thing, not a book or another baby, or doing anything else for that matter will change this fact.

Nothing can fix it. No one can make this pain go away. Somehow I'll just have to survive it. I guess I just need to find a way to live through it?

I find myself questioning will anyone even want to read a book as sad as this? Is it even worth putting my energy into, when I could be putting it elsewhere? Into my family. Into things that make me feel good?

I feel the same way about all of my work. Is it pointless? Is it a waste of my time? Does anyone even care?

I certainly don't at the moment. It all feels so frivolous. Unnecessary. Pointless. Maybe even mildly narcissistic?

Does it actually even help anyone?

(At the time I didn't realise I WAS actually writing my book as these journal entries became exactly that.)

6th April 2017

Sometimes I'm unsure
who my grief is even for.

The three babies I lost
Or the two who remain
yet have missed so much.

Do I grieve
for my babies
for my husband
for the family I imagined
for our relationship.

Or my own naivety.

7th April 2017

Every morning I think…today will be the day my motivation will
return. Then by the time I get through the essentials, you know,
feed the little people, get dressed, maintain some semblance of
normal… I'm spent.

I literally have nothing left to care about anything else. But maybe
that's okay? Maybe that's how it's meant to be. I'm trying not to
beat myself up on the days where survival is all I can manage.

10 April 2017

Things I know to be true today.

1. Running for the first time in a year bloody hurts. Everywhere.
2. It is impossible for me to think about how sad I am when I am
    running.
3. Post-running high is worth how much I intensely dislike the
    actual running part.
4. Running is excellent at shaking off 'blah' feelings.

5.   Running is a legit way to get forty minutes of not having to hear *'Muuuuuummmm I'm hungry.'*
6.   It's unlikely that I'll be able to sit down tomorrow.

11th April 2017

I feel like life used to be simple. Previously when I wanted to do something, I probably mulled over it for a minute, (maybe even less) and off I went.

Once decisions were made I mostly just kept moving. Regardless of how things turned out, I just dealt with whatever challenges came up, as they came up. I don't remember ever before questioning everything I did and why I did it.

Now I don't believe there is a single thing in my life that I haven't questioned in the last month.

Friendships.
Social outings.
The way we spend our time.
The way we spend our money.
Our relationship.
Work.
Our house.

Of course, most of it is probably because I am totally avoiding having to think about the biggest question of all.

Will we try again or are we done?

I can't even go there at the minute. That question is on the shelf. I thought this would be a complete relief. Instead it has just given me eleven-billion questions about everything else in my life.

Why am I doing this again?
Is all the time I put into this worth it?
Do I enjoy this?
What would life look and feel like if I didn't do it?
Is this right for us anymore?

Maybe a big change would help?
Maybe this is a bad time to make any changes?
Am I going crazy?

Is it good to be questioning everything in life? Or should I be just accepting what is?

Of course I don't want to wake up at 60 and realise I just did what I thought I was meant to do. Only to realise that I actually had a lot of choices that I didn't bother making.

But then again isn't acceptance, where happiness is found?

That's what I tell people in my yoga classes. Yes I'm totally questioning all that too. Feeling like a total fraud telling people to quieten their inner voices, whilst mine is going certifiably insane.

In-between all this questioning I guess I *have* been making some progress. I've slowly been working my way through my happy list.

We went away last week as a family and it was nice to have no obligations, no work, no 'should be doings'. Life is so easy on holidays, the hardest decision is 'do we eat out or buy something and eat in?'

We all like each other more. We're more patient. More connected. And then you come back to reality and everything feels like a hard slog again. Plus you've got three thousand loads of washing to catch up on.

I've been trying to keep that holiday feeling going. In particular, staying off my phone, because god knows that little 'smart' device is often the reason for my overwhelm.

I've replaced social media with lots of reading and that feels so good. Reading real books too because there really is nothing better than holding actual paper in your hands and turning real pages. Also this means there is no chance of getting distracted and 'just checking in on Facebook', and next thing you know it's an hour later…

I started working through *The Artist's Way* by Julie Cameron. I've been doing a little bit of each day and though the commitment is only to myself, it has kept me doing my own writing and creating every day rather then once a month when I actually 'have time'.

Journalling is something that I've been doing a lot of since these losses. Writing down all my crazy thoughts definitely helps and the morning pages task has been reminding me that I do better when I write daily, not just when it all gets to much and I hit rock bottom. It helps me avoid that cycle of...

I remember to do things that make me feel good.

I feel good.

I do more social things.

I get tired.

I start letting the stuff that keeps it all together go ie. eating well, not relying on caffeine, moving, writing, giving myself time to sit and feel.

I crash and burn from emotional overwhelm and feel like I'm drowning in the grief and anxiety of it all.

Yep it's a super fun cycle. One that I need to stay on top of to keep myself out of.

13th April 2017

It's Good Friday. Although it doesn't feel very good. Perhaps I'm just in a bad mood today? Why is it that any big days now just remind me of what I don't have and where we should be by now?

Easter reminds me that this time last year I felt like I had everything. I was pregnant and about to go to Bali. I had no idea how much pain was in store for us over the following 12 months.

I almost feel like that life belonged to a different person. I don't remember what it was like to feel like her anymore? This makes me sad and also a little happy, which I realise probably makes zero sense.

14th April 2017

The changing seasons
now feel like personal affronts.

Painful reminders of time passing,
forgotten dreams,
and lives not lived.

15th April 2017

I met with a good friend of mine today and she said something that really pushed my buttons. She was talking about her relationship and said something along the lines of *"I've just realised that all of these situations and events really mean nothing and I'm the only one giving them a negative meaning. So now I'm just choosing to go on with what I'm doing and not give negative meaning to meaningless things".*

Whilst she was talking entirely about her own situation and not mine, I've been thinking about this all afternoon.

Are the things that happen to us completely meaningless?

Does nothing have meaning until we assign it?

Do we create our own suffering by giving situations negative meanings?

If that's the case, can we choose to give something negative that happens to us a positive meaning?

Can it be something that makes us feel grateful, rather then completely ripped off by life?

So if that's the truth of it … Is this suffering my own creation?

Over the last year I've met a number of women who have experienced losses. All of whom say that rather than it breaking them, actually (their words) *'changed them in a positive way.'*
The experience of loss has made them more present, loving, grateful women, mothers, partners, lovers…

I keep running into this perspective everywhere. While I have moments of gratitude, I know I'm definitely not there yet. I feel like I want to interrogate these women with questions. *'But why… How?… no but seriously HOW?*

I want to know how they pushed passed the pain and unfairness of it all to give this experience the meaning a positive meaning. How have they come to not only be grateful, but where they have reconciled the fact that it was never meant to be any other way.

I'm not sure how I'll get there yet, though I feel like the path is getting clearer. I feel like I need to get to a place where the meaning of all of this is something I can live with. Where I no longer feel like I have to ask *'Why me'* because it will be *'Of course me and I'm okay with that'.*

I guess it's like any of the bad stuff we experience in life. Separation. Death. Betrayal. Loss. Divorce. Hurt. Breakdown.

It all feels like hell while we're going through it but we always seem to find a way in hindsight. We find a way to reconcile the lessons of why we had to go through it to get where we are now. We decide what it will mean to us. We find a way to create our own healing, and to make our own peace with it all.

17th April 2017

She woke each morning,
and stretched lazily.
Her hand instinctively
finding the round curve
of her centre.

Each morning gifted
a brief moment
before she remembered
the truth of her own loneliness.

19th April 2017

It drives me crazy how I can be going along okay, feeling like I'm
finally getting somewhere with my grief and then… BAM. Out of
nowhere it slams me back down. Suddenly I'm a distracted, crying
mess who can't seem to focus on anything for longer than a
minute.

That's me today.

I thought I was doing okay. I had been taking the time to do things
just for me. I had been spending time writing and creating. I had
been slowly readjusting my work so that I could feel positive again.

I had plans to do some work today and instead I've spent most of
it laying on the couch or the bed crying.

Andrew thinks I've totally lost the plot. He is not saying as much
(smart man) but I can see it in his eyes. They say *'How can you go
from where you were yesterday to here?'*

I wish I knew.

It could be hormones, I guess. Or perhaps that is just a convenient
excuse for this raging destructive feeling I have inside me.

Despite the fact that I feel like I want to run away from myself, I
know the only way past these feelings is through. So I'm going to
make myself a cuppa and do a meditation.

It's actually the last thing I want to do (sitting still and feeling this
shit) but I think it's the only thing that might actually work.

29th April

She wandered the house
unable to focus.
Every few moments
seeking distraction in something new.
Each task quickly losing its shine
as her mind inevitably wandered
back to her sadness.

She was always
shifting, moving, looking.
Busying herself in defence.
Because she knew
that in stillness
the darkness
would drag her under.

11th May 2017

I almost didn't go to counselling today. I've been feeling good. I feel lighter and happier. I feel insanely in love with my little family.

Right here and now, life feels really good.

I asked myself - *'Do I really need this?'*

Truthfully, my answer was *'No, I don't need this, but I want it.'* Unlike every other time I've been to counselling I wasn't at a breaking point. I was feeling on top of things for a change.

I wanted to make sure I wasn't just burying my hurt down so deep I couldn't feel it anymore. I've actually come to a place where I'm okay with feeling the hurt of losing these babies.* The hurt is so entangled with my feelings of love for them that I don't want to lose either. Both are important to me.

Even as I write these words I feel a little bit like - who the hell am I now? Only a few months ago, I would have been raging against a statement like that.

47

I would scoff at the disgusting positivity of it all. But now I understand. If you don't and you find yourself raging, please let yourself rage. I understand that too.

On the drive to counselling I ran scenarios in my head. I envisaged myself telling her how well I was doing and us not having much else to talk about. I also imagined the opposite scenario where she picked apart my story and showed me how I wasn't doing as well as I thought.

Very early in our conversation she explained how she felt like today was an ending. A conclusion to something, though she wasn't sure what. She looked to me for an answer but I had none. Later she mentioned that today was full moon in Scorpio and how it carries the energy of trials and tribulations and the lessons we take from it. When she went on to say '*This energy repeats again in October*' it was suddenly very clear why I was here, and what this ending was about.

It was the full moon in May 2016 when I delivered my tiny 16 week old Orion. He was meant to be due in October. *Scorpio energy.*

I've come to believe that the two losses I experienced after Orion were mostly because I hadn't dealt with my feelings of losing him. Primarily, the guilt I felt. Whether this has any bearing on my ability to carry another, I really don't have the answer to that. This is not me beating myself up for not dealing with that first loss. I don't blame the past me for what happened. In fact, I actually think it all happened exactly as it should.

All three losses were meant to bring me to this place where I feel okay with all of it. I feel ready to live again from a place of acceptance. I'm ready to surrender to all that life involves; the good and the bad, the love and the hurt, the joy and the incredibly painful.

Just before I fell pregnant this last time, I remember my mantra was '*Open my heart*', '*Open my heart*', '*Open my heart*'. I remember at the time I was intending that I wanted my heart opened to the possibility of a new baby.

Ironically the universe delivered just not in the way I had intended.

My third loss cracked my heart WIDE open. It was the most painful thing I've ever experienced and yet I find myself grateful for it. I love more deeply now. I'm more painfully aware of how fragile it all is and I want to soak it all in, not seek distraction from it.

During the energy work part of our session, our moods were both lighter than usual. Normally I don't talk and simply lie with my eyes closed. This time we chatted about life in general, hers and mine.

Then it happened.

I can only explain it as I experienced it and I'm fully aware of the woo woo factor of this explanation.

She had her hands on my belly. We were mid-conversation and we both stopped. I felt like I was suddenly in a vacuum. There was no sound. It felt almost like time stopped for a moment. And as soon as it began, it was over.

She stopped massaging my belly and said *'Wow. I don't know what that was.'*

She took a moment away from me, as if trying to gather her thoughts.

'I'm not really sure but I think that might have been a walk in.'

I had no clue what she was talking about but I knew whatever had just happened was like nothing I'd ever experienced before. I explained to her what I'd felt.

She replied *'Yep I think that a year ago, something walked in and whoever it was just walked out.'*

By now I am mildly freaking out. My entire body was covered in goosebumps.

'I don't get the feeling that this was a negative walk in.' She went on to explain that sometimes a higher being will walk in and take over. *'It felt angelic'.*

We went on to chat about this further and what it might mean. I can't tell you why (I did warn you we were headed into total woo woo territory) but this explanation feels right to me.

A year ago I gave up. It felt too hard, too much. I didn't feel like I could go on living the life I was. It wasn't that I felt suicidal in any way, but that I just couldn't do any of it anymore.

Apparently I didn't have to.

I walked out of that counselling session feeling lighter, and for the first time in a long time more like myself. Not necessarily the me that I was before all of this happened, but a wiser, stronger version. I immediately wanted to cut all of my hair back off to my short pixie cut, which I suddenly realised I'd been growing for exactly a year.

14th May 2017

Mother's Day.

Today holds mixed feelings for me now. To hold both grief and immense joy and gratitude in your heart at the same time is a superpower of Mother's everywhere.

We don't just grieve for our babies' lost. We also grieve for our tiny babies who disappear as they grow into children and then adults. Every new stage is also a loss of something that once was. All of it a lesson in letting go gracefully to embrace something new.

13th June 2017

I've been reading back over my journalling from the past year. I wish I could go back to the start of the year and tell myself to surrender to it all and stop pushing so hard in every area of my life.

But maybe that's why I had to go through it - to learn total surrender.

I was doing so much. I was giving my energy away to so many things and people in my life. It's unsurprising that I ended up so depleted and run down. Not an ideal way to grow a baby.

I know when we start trying again I will focus only on growing a healthy baby and loving my little family. I will protect my energy instead of giving more of it to others than I give to myself.

Exquisite self care starts now.

What does that look like for me?

+ nourishing food and lots of water
+ positive self talk
+ daily movement
+ daily journalling
+ daily stillness / meditation
+ daily oil self-massage

14th June 2017

A friend told me she is pregnant today. Again. *Accidentally.*

I am ragingly jealous.

It hurt even more because her words were...

'Holy shit'
'What am I going to do?'
'I've only just got my body back - this wasn't supposed to happen now.'

It made me mad to hear but I also felt mad at myself for not speaking up in that moment and saying...

'I don't want to hear this. It hurts too much.'

Why did I put her feelings before my own? Why am I still putting everyone else before myself?

Then just because the world is testing me today. Another friend gave birth. *To twins.*

My period is also due any minute which makes this the trifecta of shitty days.

16th June 2017

Where did you go when you left?
I still feel you here,
some days.

Whenever I start to question
you show me a sign,
a little reminder of you.

I prayed
and you spoke to me,
but I couldn't tell your voice from my own.

17th June 2017

Life has continued ticking on. I feel like I've stopped spinning my wheels and once again I'm moving forward.

I've started having regular rebirthing sessions which sounds totally hippy and woo but is quite simply profound and profoundly simple all at the same time. One of the women who comes to my yoga studio facilities them weekly for myself and a couple of other friends. We simply breathe for a hour or two and then share what comes up for a us at the end.

The breath is a little different than what we practice in yoga. In rebirthing we breathe in a circular way. Each inhale leans into the exhale and the exhale leans into the next inhale and on it goes.

The idea is that the breath works on a cellular level and helps you to bring up and release old memories, emotions and experiences that you've stuffed down deep and didn't (or couldn't) process. Like always, I went into it open-heartedly skeptical and walked out of our first session filled with gratitude.

The funny thing is once you've released the memories, it's very hard to remember what they were or feel the emotion of them anymore. So while I'm going to try and describe some of the things that have happened in our sessions I really have quite a sketchy memory around them.

During our first session I had the intense feeling of energy moving from my belly to my heart as I breathed in, and from my heart to my belly as I breathed out. I can't tell you why or how, but I felt like this was something I needed to do to let my babies go. Or maybe not let go entirely, but move them to a space where I can love them for what they are rather than for who and what I wish they'd been.

While I was breathing I remember hearing *'trust'* and *'cradled'* over and over again.

Afterwards we journal or draw an oracle card.

I found myself writing:

'I am held. I have never been more held than when I hold myself'.

And also:

'It's time to stop being half in. Stop trying to protect yourself from feeling by staying stuck in past emotions or by pre-empting the worst. Life is about all of it. The good. The bad. The painful. The joyful. You can't pick and choose and you don't want to.'

The oracle card I drew simply said: *'Hello from heaven.'*

Hello indeed.

20th June 2017

I was listening to a podcast the other day with Brene Browne and she was talking about this concept of the 'darkest teacher'. It was spot on.

We all have a dark teacher - an experience in our life that sucks... HARD.

Something we feel like we barely survived and yet when we find ourselves on the other side of it, we realise that actually the whole experience taught us more about ourselves and the world than anything else before it.

Obviously no one is putting their hands up to go through any of the shitty experiences of their lives again, but hopefully with a little hindsight we can see that there was something positive that came out of them anyway. Perhaps even, dare I say it, our darkest teacher was an experience that we needed to go through, to learn the things we needed to learn.

Dark teachers come many different forms – losing a job, death, illness, breaking up, breaking down, losing a whole lot of money, fire, stuffing up, a verbal or physical fight, a car accident, losing a baby.

Our darkest teacher stops us dead in our tracks.

It puts the brakes on in every areas of our lives because suddenly we're in survival mode and all our energy is used up simply getting through the day.

BUT what if this forced STOP was actually an invitation.

What if this horrible, shitty, unfair experience that really shouldn't be a happening to a nice person like you, was an invitation from the universe to WAKE UP, to pay attention.

What if this whole experience was happening because you're being invited to...

… turn and pivot in some area of your life that you'd become stuck in.

… build your boundaries and to stop letting others walk all over you.

… get really clear about what you want to be doing with your life and what you *don't* want to be doing

… recognise how fragile life is and how lucky you are to be living it

… realise how toxic someone in your life is and why you need to let them go

… start giving yourself the love and attention you deserve

… stop wasting your days doing stuff that makes you feel like crap

… look after your body rather than waiting until it falls apart to do something

… actually recognise and FEEL how good your life already is, right now, without all of those things you've been feeling so desperate for

… notice how much support you have around you

… love the people in your life better

… rest more

… stop rushing through your life

… stress less and enjoy more

What happens if we survive our darkest teacher but don't take the invitation?

We're presented with another opportunity, another invitation.

Perhaps we find the EXACT same thing seems to happen over and over and over again.

Until finally we take the invitation. We follow the message we're being given.

It's why we seem to repeat the same patterns in our lives until finally we say ENOUGH!

I'm done. I've learned.

And on we live.

24th June 2017

We're up at Noosa without the kids for a couple of nights while the boys stay with their Aunty. I honestly don't know how I would survive life without her.

It occurred to me on the way up that this is the first time I've truly been without kids since before I was pregnant with Eamon. This is a very strange feeling. I went away for a night once when I was pregnant with Rory and once when I was pregnant with the second baby I lost.

But right now, there is no one but us.

I know that this time is important for us to have, but it is hard all the same.

I feel like I've been asleep for most of last year. I know I was present for it but clearly my brain was somewhere else. I don't want to live like that anymore.

26th June 2017

There are moments
where she feels happiness rise up
in her throat like foam.

It bubbles out of her as laughter,
endless chatter,
unconscious movement.

But then she remembers,
and guilt follows in his absence.

29th June 2017

MTHFR FUCKER

I've just been to my GP today and I am so flipping angry. I went to
pick up results from tests my naturopath requested.

As she printed off the results she said *'It all looks pretty good except for
your iron and calcium levels.'*

But we already knew that. I took my results and headed home. It
wasn't until I got home and started having a closer look that I read
that the gene mutation MTHFR was present.

I don't know about you but a mutated gene felt somewhat relevant
so I went to dreaded Dr Google and investigated a bit further. I
freaked out as common issues related to a MTHFR are recurrent
miscarriages and genetic complications. There are actual support
groups for this thing!

I calmed down to read on. My version of the mutation is
considered a minor issue and means that the way my body
processes Folate and B vitamins is somewhat impaired and not
completely broken. Suggested treatment is making sure you are
eating a diet full of natural folate and B vitamins and/or
supplementing to make sure there is no deficit.

Okay, is it just me or would you not think that to be a relevant
thing for a doctor to tell you if you've experienced genetic
complications and multiple miscarriages?

I can't even. This whole process has me losing faith in the Western
medical system. I get it. You can't prescribe me any medication for

this particular issue. But surely an explanation of what it means for my body would have been somewhat helpful given you're the one with the 8 year degree, not me.

Although I'm thoroughly pissed off, I also feel somewhat relieved. I don't believe this is THE answer, but I believe it is one part of the whole. I'm coming to see how infertility is a like big jigsaw puzzle of tiny little pieces and they all need to fit together in a certain way for a healthy baby to be born. (I'm also realising how much we're all amazing little miracles who overcame ridiculously bad odds to be here).

Given the fact that my first loss was just over 15 months after I'd had Rory and only a month or so after I stopped breastfeeding. I think it's probably safe to say my body was in a deficit at that point.

Then for the following two losses, not much had changed other than I was now not only struggling to look after myself, I was grieving, highly wired and anxious about my whether I would lose another baby. Not exactly a healthy environment to grow a baby.

This to me feels true.

I need to take better care of my body through the food I put in it, how regularly I move it and how often I rest.

I need to slow down and manage my stress.

I need to trust that my body, mind and spirit can heal and that I will have another healthy baby.

30th June 2017

Today is the due date for my second baby I lost.

Strangely I feel okay. I wasn't counting down the days like I did with Orion. Although writing that does make me feel somewhat guilty. Should I still be counting down the days?

There is no right way is there? Feel shitty if you do and shitty if you don't.

I actually feel somewhat at peace with it all now. I'm not sure if it's the rebirthing. Or all the writing it out I've been doing every morning. Or the meditation. But I truly feel okay with it all.

I feel excited about the prospect of trying again. It doesn't fill me with dread anymore.

I feel like I know myself better than ever through all of this. I'm in a really good place.

1st July 2017

After trudging around for many months
with her head down.

She looked around
to realise.

Life was not as dark
as she'd been imagining.

2nd July 2017

I don't think I'd realised how stressful trying for another baby had become until we decided to go on a break. It's been about four months now since our last loss and I honestly feel like a different person.

I sleep better.

I don't feel like I'm in a constant state of panic.

I've given myself a big ol' break in so many areas of my life that when I look back I'm not surprised my body (or mind, or emotions, or spirit) weren't ready.

Rory was only one when we experienced our first traumatic loss at 16 weeks and then we went straight into trying to have another baby. And then we lost another. Then another.

Looking back I think I must have been a little crazy.

At the time, I thought trying again was the answer. But now I can see how important healing time actually is.

It's given me a whole new perspective on the whole process. It's given me so much respect for how our bodies actually work. It's given us a chance to be partners / friends / lovers again without grief or trying for a baby between us.

If you've been trying to conceive for any period of time – you know how stressful and emotional the whole experience can be.

It's also incredibly lonely. Sure, you may have connected with the countless other women in online forums but in the real world, it probably feels like no one understands what you're going through.

'Relax' they tell you. 'It will happen when it's meant to happen.'

They don't get the manic counting of days and dates. The obsessive tracking of every sign in your body. Looking for clues that you're ovulating, implantation, possibly, nervously, tentatively, pregnant.

This approach to trying to conceive is exhausting.

In many way your friends are right, you do need to relax. But if one more person tells you that, you might just rip their heads off.

How do you relax when something you want so badly just isn't happening? When something you've always dreamed of seems to be happening to everyone else but you.

Doing nothing feels counterproductive. How will relaxing help you to do anything?

So you turn to the internet and Dr. Google gives you a barrage of things you're doing wrong.

Suddenly you need to:

- Change your diet.
- Stop drinking coffee
- Drink more water
- Move more
- Move less
- Sleep more.
- Take supplements.
- Have more sex.
- Have less sex.
- Have sex at a precise time of day, on the right day of your cycle, in the right position while standing on your head. (Okay so maybe that's a slight exaggeration.)

It's not surprising that you're anything but relaxed. It feels like there is no time to relax because you've got so many parts of your life that you need to change before you get pregnant.

This is all before you even start down any roads that involve fertility specialists and treatments.

I know it feels counter intuitive but I honestly believe the answer is you need to stop. Take a deep breath. Stand back a little.
How does the stress of all of this feel in your body?

Tight.
Restrictive.
Panicky.
It feels like you have no room to move.

You're probably rushing from thing to thing. Every single moment is filled with thoughts and plans to do more, to make sure you get pregnant this month.

But all this is doing is telling your body that life is too stressful. And your body won't create new life where it believes it can't be sustained.

Rather than focusing on all the things you absolutely must do or else you'll never get your baby. I think we need to focus instead on making ourselves feel good.

Focus on your health and being in the best health you can, without the pressure of *'If I eat this I'll never conceive'*. Continue to do and plan things based on things that make you happy, rather than on whether or not you might be pregnant or not by then.

At the end of the year, you'll either be pregnant, or you won't.

I know I'd rather spend that time looking after myself instead of stressing about doing everything wrong.

I know I'd rather continue living and enjoying my life rather than putting everything on hold while I focus on trying to conceive.

I know how I'd rather feel.

14th July 2017

I had the most amazing rebirthing session today. I felt like I was present for my D&Cs. Like I was actually there for everything that happened. Awake and conscious.

I'd never thought about it before but we experience this traumatic procedure and we are not even present for it. It's unsurprising that we have trouble dealing with the trauma of something we're unconscious for.

During our session today I re-lived the freezing cold of the surgical theatre. I could feel the oxygen mask on my face and the rough way they were pressing it into my cheeks because I was mildly freaking out.

I was aware of the doctors and nurses moving around me. But I didn't feel afraid. I felt supported because **I could feel three little sets of hands holding me.**

They were with me the whole time. Nothing overly dramatic happened medically. It was all very calm and ordered but that feeling of not being alone will always be with me.

They were there all along.

15th July 2017

Day 1 of my cycle. Even though we weren't even trying this month I still feel that particular heavy sadness of my period arriving.

I'm afraid it will be a really long road to our 3rd baby. What if it takes another 2 or 3 or 4 or 5 years? Or more?

How will I survive that?

While I know the answer is the same way I already have. By grieving, by reaching out for support, by letting everything else fall alway, by taking it day by day, hour by hour. My mind still jumps in with the question.

'But how will I survive that again?'

My heart knows I can, but my brain is not so sure. I guess the only way to know is to try.

I wish there was some way to be certain that I wouldn't have to go through another loss. But that's all of life, isn't it? You have to open yourself up to the possibility of being hurt if you want to open yourself up to more love.

I don't think the connection is ever more obvious than to a mother who is trying to have a baby after multiple losses.

The risk feels so close I can feel the heat of it before I even try.

I really don't want to feel or live that way. I want to be open to life and love, whatever the risk of being hurt.

Our baby is worth it.

6th August 2017

This path feels like two steps forwards one step back. Last week I was definitely stepping back. I was incredibly emotional for no particular reason other than 'everything'. I just wanted to cry from the sadness of it all. I also felt incredibly pissed off at the world in general.

I tried all of my usual tricks to shake the heaviness. Journalling. Meditation. Yoga. Walking. Talking. Nothing was shaking it.

So I booked in to see my counsellor who I hadn't seen for months. We spoke about my anxiety, which I didn't even realise I had until a couple of months ago. Now I know what that feeling is, I look back and think I've been suffering it for most of my life. I've just never had a name for that tight racing feeling in my chest or the heat in my belly. Because I've never known what it was I've never really expressed it or dealt with it.

It's funny how this whole path has made me learn so much more about myself. Not just about now, but also things that happened years ago.

I am so much more in tune with what's going on for me but in all honesty sometimes that also feels painful. Denial and numbing sometimes seem easier to deal with.

One part of me wishes I could just go back to who I was before all of this. Before I lost at all. I miss being her. I didn't realise it then, but life was easier. It was easy because I wasn't really seeing all of it. I was completely in denial about death and its presence in all of our lives. I was living as if death was a distant possibility, rather than something that is a present reality for all of us, at all times.

I know the concept of death can be a gift. It's a pretty special person who can live a full life with constant knowledge that today could be the very last day for all of us. But how do you live with that knowledge and keep a joyful heart? How do you live and love without being sad about the inevitability of loss?

It's something I'm definitely struggling with at the moment. I feel like I'm on the cusp of something but I can feel myself holding back. I'm not sure I want to go through this veil and onto the other side. It feels scary and vulnerable and I'm not sure I'm ready to live like that yet.

14th August 2017

I've just spent my birthday weekend at a yoga for trauma teacher training. This pretty accurately sums up the lighthearted state of my life at the moment.

It was both amazing and not at all what I expected. It definitely confirmed what I've already felt about trauma; that you can't heal anyone but yourself. You can learn tools and resources to work towards healing, but ultimately it comes down to you.

I found it interesting to learn though that sharing your story is considered an important part of healing. Which I guess just further emphasises why I feel writing about my losses has been such an important part of healing for me.

16th August 2017

I have this distinct memory from the middle of last year. I was talking about anxiety with someone I was working with, who also happens to be a close friend. She was sharing her experience with it and she asked if I'd ever felt it.

I said no and 100% believed that to be the truth.

Ironically looking back, my anxiety at that point was at peak level.

I've always considered myself to be a pretty calm and relaxed sort of person. And I am... on the outside. But I've come to realise only recently how much I internalise. I literally stress inwardly and never realised that anxiety isn't something you do, rather something you feel.

The things that started to unravel anxiety for me

- My naturopath gave me this herbal mixture (I fondly call sludge) for my nervous system and I could literally feel it calming my body down.

- I've been making time to write and meditate daily and I now notice that on the days I don't, I feel tight and stress-y in my chest.

- A long conversation with my counsellor brought up the fact that I never really show anger. Instead I bury that feeling inside, which made me start to question... what else am I burying?

- A rebirthing session the other week was actually physically painful as my body released 30+ years of stuff I've been holding. Afterwards I sobbed for the sadness of it all. The next day I woke up pissed off with life and everyone in it.

- Though I was hesitant at first, (the needles freaked me out) acupuncture has literally been melting my anxiety away. I'm so zen afterwards I can barely form sentences.

- I've noticed that Eamon (my eldest) can be quite anxious about things, especially when it comes to school or social situations with people he doesn't know well. Unlike me, he is excellent at voicing how he is feeling. I'm doing my very best to not teach him to silence that voice.

- It wasn't until I came down from my super anxious state that I could actually even feel and recognise anxiety in my body. I had to give up coffee (sob!) and get honest with myself about the fact that it just creates more anxiety in my body. It makes me feel restless and unsettled, like I constantly need to do more or something bad will happen.

- My anxiety gets worse when I let life get too busy. If I don't have space to do nothing I can feel it starting to build in my body and my mind starts racing. It's like I can't catch a single thought.

What I'm doing to manage my anxiety.

A morning routine.

I know I feel better if I write and meditate every day and the only way this happens is if I get up before everyone else to do it. It doesn't always work and sometimes Rory joins me, but it's definitely helping. (Speak of the devil, Rory has just arrived on the couch next to me as I type this. It's 5.40am, dark and cold. I've already meditated, written in my journal and done some really gentle yoga. It feels like I'm already winning the day).

Being more mindful of food.

It's funny I've spent most of my life looking at food from the perspective of *'Will this make me fat, or not'*.

(Actually that's not really funny at all, is it? I feel quite sad that I've wasted so long feeling this way).

Now I ask *'How will this make me feel?'* Caffeine was the first to go. Gluten also makes me feel yuck. I think it might also be time to break up with my beloved red wine.

Support

Once upon a time I didn't even go to the Doctor when I was sick. Now I regularly visit a naturopath, acupuncturist, counsellor and have rebirthing sessions weekly.

I turned off the noise.

I have a love/ hate relationship with social media. I still use it but I needed it to not be in every minute of my every day. So I'm trying to be a lot more mindful of scrolling.

Instead, I try to ask before I go into Facebook or Instagram *'What am I going here for?'* and then only doing that one thing rather than being lost in the black hole. But its not just social media that was creating noise for me.

Podcasts and audiobooks were also filling up my brain and every spare minute – so I'm trying to stick to fiction instead. I'm trying to read and listen for enjoyment rather than constant learning.

Time for 'pointless' creativity.

I'm always creating, but I'd forgotten how to create without a purpose. There was always a reason to it – whether that was for the blog, to share on social or even just something to give to a friend.

I'd forgotten how good creativity is when there is absolutely no point to it. I've been trying to make time each week for more of this. At the minute I'm getting back into jewellery making (my 10 year old self is loving this) and teaching myself to write with brush pens.

17th August 2017

I asked Andrew last night whether he was ready to start trying again and he is definitely still undecided. He says he just wants me to be absolutely ready. But what does that actually look like?

I know I want to go into trying again with all the positivity I had with Eamon and Rory. I want the excitement and daydreaming. Of course, I know I will still have to play it day by day. But really that's all anyone ever gets. They just don't realise it.

My body is healthy and cycling regularly. I feel like I have a lot of resources now to deal with my anxiety.

On the other hand, I also don't want to speed ahead. I don't want to rush it. I want right now too. Just the four of us.

22nd August

I want life to be simple.

Is it up to me to just make that decision?

Life IS simple. Just like that?

I've realised that I overcomplicate so much of my life with overthinking, re-playing, over-worrying, anxiety.

Like my Grandma said a few weeks ago when she visited my home for the first time.

I have two beautiful boys.
I have a great man.
I have a lovely home.

Don't I have everything?

Why then can I not let go of this idea of a third baby?

I think it's okay to want more as long as my happiness doesn't depend on them. I don't think it does anymore.

26th August 2017

I'm trying to lighten up more. I don't even know why I stress so much. I remember I used to even stress about going somewhere with both boys. I would spend so much time imagining how it was going to play out. Creating all the scenarios in my head instead of just showing up for whatever happened. Stress would pile on top of stress.

Everything in our lives had started to feel like an event to be endured rather than something to be enjoyed. I remember having this feeling about our holiday to Bali. I spent so much time stressing and worrying about all the things that could go wrong. What a terrible way to live.

While I feel a looooonng way away from this type of thinking now, I also know it's not hard to fall back into. It's only a simple mindset shift after all.

I know I need to keep myself grounded in this when we eventually start trying again. How?

Writing
Meditation
Self-massage
Baths
Staying focused on fun and enjoyment
Movement to shake out the negative energy.

3rd September 2017

Part of me wants to go back to being unconscious. I don't want the pressure of 'doing it right' all the time.

I just want to do my best and be content with that. I know that's my choice to make but it feels so hard to do.

I've always been a planner. Being future focused used to make me happy. Now it doesn't. It's like the mirage has been broken and I see it for what it really is.

So unknown, so unpredictable.

10th September 2017

This last week has been horrible. Other than Wednesday where I dragged myself out of bed for work, I've pretty much been in agony with body aches and fevers. That then turned into an ear infection which made me want to crawl out of my own body.

It has definitely made me appreciate my health though. I didn't know how good I felt until I didn't.

I also had the thought when I was feeling my worst - *'Why do I want a third child?'* I have two beautiful boys. Why would I go and complicate that when we are just coming out the other side of baby-land.

Rory is only just emerging from being a baby himself and I'm really enjoying their ages at the minute. Possibly more than I ever have.

I feel like they've both missed a lot from me in the last year. Do they even remember when I was happy?

I feel like the last 6 months have been the first time in a long time where I've just enjoyed our little family. I've finally dropped the constant feeling like I need to do more, achieve more. I've just been here. Living. Loving them. Enjoying what is.

13th September 2017

Day 1 of my cycle. A fresh start. I have a feeling this cycle is going to be a good one. I've only got a few pages left in my journal. It's crazy how different life is now from my very first entry. Back then I was pregnant, highly anxious and spiralling down. Now I feel so much more content with my life. I feel like I've accepted the whole messy lot of it.

I'm ready for the reality that trying again may mean another loss but I know I want to try again anyway.

What I will do differently this time:

+ only tell a couple of people (reserve my energy for growing our baby)
+ meditation, reading, rest
+ supplements, keep eating really well
+ stay positive and be excited
+ talk to the baby, connect right from the start
+ focus on gratitude
+ keep living my happy life

6th October 2017

I decided to quit everything this week. The last few months have been full of weekly acupuncture, taking all the supplements, doing all the right things, blood tests and tracking my cycle.

Basically doing everything but what I want to be doing which is starting trying to conceive again.

I've been waiting to get the green light from my acupuncturist, my naturopath, my GP, someone, basically anyone. Almost as if someone was going to issue me a free pass, a sure thing that my next pregnancy will become a baby in my arms.

My anxiety had started creeping back in a big way and I could feel my obsession with getting everything just perfect (and feeling the inevitable frustration when it wasn't.)

I decided it was time to stop.

Not everything entirely. But all the things I've been doing because I think I should.

I'm still going to take my supplements and Chinese herbs because I feel better on them. I'm still going to keep eating way more red meat than I would usually choose to because my iron levels are still low. I know I'll keep eating how I have been because it gives me so much more energy.

But otherwise I need to just stop and trust.

Nothing can guarantee us that the next pregnancy, nor any pregnancy, will work out. But I know in my heart that I'm ready to try again.

I don't want to do this in an obsessed stressful way.

I don't want to be tracking and charting and timing when we have sex.

I don't want to have to worry about that one glass of red wine that I had last week and whether it affected our chances of falling pregnant.

I just want to stop *stopping* pregnancy happening and let my body (and the universe) decide when it's the right time.

I said this to Andrew the other day after an acupuncture appointment because I'd come home feeling like I was still doing everything wrong. I felt like I was STILL broken.

He reminded me how much I'm doing right. I'm doing 1000 times better at looking after myself than when we were trying last year. I have to trust that we are both healthy and it will work out.

Trust when you've been badly burned is so incredibly hard. But I do believe it's the only way I'm going to be able to be brave enough to go back into this particular fire.

8th October 2017

I feel so tired today. I ran my women's circle last night on relationships and as always the exact right combination of people showed up for it. I went out for dessert afterwards with a couple of girlfriends and I just feel so damn grateful for my life.

Without intending to, my morning pages have become focused on what I'm calling in. Each morning I'll write a free-for-all for a page or so, then switch to a list of things I'm grateful for and end with what I'm calling in.

It's funny. It's almost like whatever I write it down I no longer have to think or obsess about. I can trust that it's there and something I'm working towards without actually having to hold so tightly or do anything about it.

Today I wrote.

I am grateful for:

1. Rory and his funny little personality. Tonight he put a basket on his head at bedtime and said *'I hiding Mummy'*. I have no idea why I found that so funny but it feels so good to be able to feel the joy of these small things again.

2. Eamon and how it often feels like he is older than me with the wisdom that comes out of his mouth.

3. Andrew and the way he supports all of my crazy ideas.

I'm calling in:

1. The soul of our baby. I'm ready to carry and birth our healthy 3rd child.

2. A close circle of friends.

3. The women who need the work that I share.

15th October

I did a test this morning. I don't know why I thought today was a good time. I'm forgiving myself for it though. I'm promising myself I will tread lightly with myself this time.

I feel sad that I'm not pregnant, although I am still feeling that glimmer of hope. Maybe I just tested too soon? I wish I'd waited the full 14 days after when I know I ovulated so that at least I'd know for sure. But I just couldn't wait.

18th October

I peed on a stick this morning. Then went about doing my makeup and getting ready for work like this is a regular, normal everyday thing to do.

The faintest second little line appeared. For a while I sat there questioning whether perhaps I was just so hopeful and wanting to be pregnant that I had now taken to imagining things.

But nope. There it is.

I looked down at my belly and said a tentative 'Hello'.

I feel surprised, even though I've been calling down this little soul every night before I fall asleep. It's become such a normal part of my day that I forget that for most people this is definitely not a normal thing to do before one falls asleep. It's like a silent prayer I say to the universe every night.

These prayers are different from those prayers of desperation I used to recite in the early days after our losses. Back then I wanted our baby immediately, right now, yesterday if possible. Then, my prayers came from a place of hurt and wanting that hurt to stop.

But more recently, my prayers have come from a different place. I feel really content with what life looks like right now. Now my prayers come from a place of knowing that there is another little soul for our family - without trying to force the how and when he or she comes to us.

There is a lot of ease to be found in trusting. It's like you can hand over your fears to someone or something else because it's not in your hands.

I guess for those who have a religion this is what that feels like, being able to trust in a god and that what will happen will happen. I guess my faith is similar, except there is no single god, just a universe that is working for us, with us, not against us.

I don't know if these two pink lines will be my baby. Either way, I'm choosing to trust that he or she is coming.

20th October

I trust.
In divine timing.
Everything unfolds as it should.
I let go of my need to push
to make things happen.

I move in the right direction with ease.
My only job is to look after myself well
To keep my mind calm and clear.

I only need to focus on one moment at a time.
This one.

Breathing into my belly.
I breathe my anxiety away.

Feeling grateful for everything
I already have.

22nd October

4 weeks and 2 days

Time is creeping at the moment. Is it because I would like to press fast forward and end up in late December? Or is it because I am doing my best to stay really present here and now where I am a mother of two and newly pregnant? Where everything is still full of hope and possibility.

I shouldn't complain. I always feel like time goes too fast so I should embrace this season of slow. I'm doing my best to rest and focus on keeping my anxiety low. I feel like I'm always on the lookout, trying to stay away from getting caught in an anxiety spiral, especially one I'm not aware of. But perhaps I'm past that?

I'm calling in:

1. The bravery to stay calm throughout this pregnancy and open up my heart despite the chance of getting hurt.

2. The health and strength to carry, grow and birth this baby.

3. Trust that this is all going to be okay.

4. The presence to be here and now for my boys, Andrew and myself.

23rd October 2017

Dear Baby,

Hello my darling.

I can't even begin to tell you how happy I am that you're here. I am doing everything I can to help you grow that healthy little body of yours. So don't you worry about a thing.

We can't wait to meet you. I think your brothers already know about you even though I haven't told them yet.

They're pretty intuitive though. I have a feeling you will be too.

I already love you so much and I'm so grateful that you chose me to be your Mama.

Love, Mum.

25th October 2017

I woke up this morning feeling nervous and excited and I'm not really sure why.

I did decide before I fell asleep last night that I wanted to feel excited about being pregnant. Surely it doesn't just happen like that? Surely it wasn't just my decision to make all along?

I decided that if we have to go through everything again I want the full experience of all of it - the good and the bad.

There is no escaping the hard parts, so why would I deny myself the good bits (like being excited) by starting this pregnancy being so anxious that I don't get to enjoy any of it.

I am excited to see this healthy baby on the first scan.

I am excited to tell the boys they are going to have a baby sister or brother.

I am excited to plan how I will tell Andrew.

I am excited about how I will tell my Mum and my sisters.

I am excited to set up the baby's room again.

I am excited to watch my belly grow big and round.

I am excited for birth.

I am excited for that first moment where you draw them up to your naked chest.

I am excited to breastfeed again.

I am excited to be a family of five.

I am excited to be pregnant.

29th October 2017

I'm enjoying keeping this secret to myself. It feel like it's this little piece of magic that I don't have to share with anyone yet. I do wonder how long I'll be able to stay this way though. My body clearly remembers how to fill out for pregnancy and is doing it fast.

Some days I forget I'm pregnant for a little while and then it's like a lovely surprise all over again when I remember. It's the exact opposite to how I felt after losing Orion. I would forget for a while that I had lost him and then suddenly that searing pain of remembering again would hit me.

I want to keep this pregnancy to ourselves until we've got the results back from the harmony test. I don't want to be fielding questions or even dealing with anyone else's energy on that until after I've made it through the two weeks of waiting for the test results.

It will be hard enough dealing with my own anxiety during this time without having to worry about others.

30th October 2017

5 weeks and 2 days

I went to the toilet this morning and there was a little colour when I went to wipe. I won't say blood but it was definitely a brown colour.

I'm trying so hard not to jump immediately to the negative but it's really challenging. Is this a sign I need to rest more? I don't think I've been doing too much?

My belly is bloated and cramping a little.

I'm just trying to breathe and not let anxiety take over.

I'm rolling this affirmation around and around in my head right now.

'I let go of my need to know what's happening. I trust that my body is strong and healthy. I am growing a healthy baby.'

31st October 2017

So yesterday seems to have been nothing after all. There was no more spotting, though I didn't do much for the rest of the day.

I still feel torn between making mental plans for this baby and trying to not get ahead of myself.

My exhaustion feels heavy and thick at the minute. I'm not sure if this is just normal first trimester exhaustion or if it is from the added fact that I feel like I'm battling to keep anxiety down most of the time as well.

Perhaps I've not worded that right. It's not a battle. I don't feel stressed and worn out doing it, although I'm sure a lot of my energy is going to breathing it away and constantly repeating my mantras to myself. It does require all of my focus. I need to be aware of my anxiety so that it doesn't take over me.

November 5th 2017

My anxiety raged today. I'm not sure if it was the comedown from the last few months or the fact that I've let some of my practices slip (meditation and yoga has been lacking in all the busy-ness lately).

The worst part of anxiety is that I find when I'm stuck in it, I'm so exhausted from carrying it that I struggle to do the things I need to do to get myself out of it. It becomes a negative cycle of being too tired to make myself feel better, so I lay around and scroll social media, which fuels the anxiety and on and on it goes.
I gave myself a bit of a pep talk today and walked slowly and without purpose to the beach. As soon as I saw the yellow flowers I knew.

I'd missed the anniversary of Orion's due date. I'd been so busy that one year since we scattered his ashes amongst the flowers had already passed. A part of me felt sad to have missed it. The rest of me cried grateful tears that I was no longer logging dates, counting the days since we'd lost him or calculating how many milestones we should have had by now.

I knew then that my anxiety was coming from those emotions I hadn't been making time for. I'd been so busy that they were being buried, which inevitably means they pop out later in ways that I often feel like I can't explain. Feeling dread about going to work, even though that's something that I really enjoy. Anger over something that would normally not worry me at all.

I sat amongst the flowers and listened to a guided meditation on surrender. Tears poured down my face as I sent a silent apology to Orion for missing his important date. I left with a weight lifted, and walked slowly home to the arms of my boys.

29th November

9 weeks!

I feel like this time is different. Although maybe I wrote that last time too?

I do feel different though. My boobs are bigger and hurt more. The sickness is worse and building. My belly is solid and I'm SO protective of it. I hate anyone touching it.

I think everything is going to be okay.

1st December 2017

We had our ten week scan today! There was a beautiful beating heart and bub was measuring exactly what I thought he/she would be.

I've also had the genetic blood test done to check for any issues.

And now we wait...

6th December 2017

Let's be honest.

No matter how much we profess to being okay with waiting, it actually really sucks.

We wait anxiously to fall pregnant.
We wait nervously for babies to arrive.
We wait fearfully for test results, when a life literally hangs in the balance.
We wait angrily for our partners to get home, when we're mad that they went out in the first place.
We wait excitedly for our big business idea to finally take off.
We wait for a distant friend to finally call us back.
We wait desperately for life to become a little less hard.
We wait for money to not be so tight.
We wait for children to grow.
We wait
We wait
We wait...

It is depressing when you feel like your life is forever on hold.

It feels like you have no control over what is happening and where it's going.

It feels scary and stressful. That negative kind of stress that you can't do anything about. You mull over it and roll scenarios around in your head hoping for it to be the right one, but always secretly imagining the worst.

You slip into talking about one day, someday, when, if...

This is not a fun place to be at all.

This place of waiting is filled with all the negative self-talk. It must be your fault, right?

That of course, can be the only explanation. **You.** The problem must be you.

From there its a slippery slope into victim-ville where you feel powerless to change anything and so ... you wait some more.

But there is a better way.

You can wake up and realise you do have control. Not of how life unfolds, but of how you feel about what does. Of how you react to what happens. You can choose to be active in the periods of waiting.

Enjoy the downtime when you're waiting for something big.

Amp up your self-love and make sure you go into whatever adventure you're waiting for full up, rather than depleted from the stress and anxiety of worrying about whether the waiting would end.

Use the waiting to clear the clutter from your life. Clean up the crap from your house, your car, your body, your heart and mind.

Make space for whatever it is you're waiting for.

Want to make more money? Get the finances you have now in order, rather than waiting until you make it big.

Want a new relationship? Do you have room in your life for one or have you filled it up with work, and social events and anything to keep yourself so busy that you don't have to think about the missing relationship. Make space so they can come in.

Want more love? Make the space to give it to yourself. It can't come in if you are so busy hating on yourself with that little internal voice.

Waiting for a baby? Channel that nurturing mama energy into yourself. Look after yourself as well as you would a child, after all you will become their home for a short while.

If we amp up the positive self-talk and loving actions towards ourself, we fill up. We become self-assured and less doubtful. We get to a place where we know that while we're still waiting, we are also okay, here, today.

We become less crazed and desperate in our waiting, and more content and open to whatever happens.

We're all waiting for something... I choose to be grateful to be doing so.

13th December 2017

We got our results back today.

Our baby passed with flying colours! No sign of any genetic issues.

And... we're having another boy!

I can't even explain how I feel.

Relieved.
Emotional.
A little disbelief.

Still mildly anxious.

I wonder if I'll ever full relax until he is in my arms? I'm going to work really hard to try to.

31st December 2017

Dear 2017,

Thank you, you big, ugly, hairy, beautiful year for...

+ showing me that I can survive more pain than I ever knew possible and still find happiness and light on the other side

+ opening my eyes to the absolutely miracle that is my two beautiful boys. I of course loved and cherished them before, but there is something about loss that has definitely opened my eyes to how we're all just bloody walking miracles. Do you know how many odds we have to overcome to even be here? I won't bore you with the stats, because lord knows my brain is filled with too many of them. Just know you're also a miracle.

+ the breakdowns that brought Andrew and I closer than ever before.

+ making me completely re-evalaute how I spend my time and helping me to realise it's my job to make time for the important things. It's okay to say a big, guilt-free NO to the things that aren't my top priorities (even when this means disappointing people I care about, which feels really hard when you're a recovering people pleaser)

+ helping me see that getting help in all kinds of places is actually being strong. It's not weak to need help to care for yourself, as I think I may have subconsciously thought previously. Naturopathy, acupuncture, counselling, energy work, rebirthing – allllll the things I now have in my toolbox for whenever I need help again.

+ connecting me with so many strong, amazing women this year. It's funny (actually it's not funny at all) how many people come out and share their stories with you when you literally bleed your heart all over a blog. I couldn't have made it through the hardest of times without these women helping me feel less alone and showing me that getting to the other side can be done.

+ delivering new ideas into my brain at 2am and then getting me going on renovations before I had the chance to talk myself out of the big scary project that is opening your own in-real-life yoga studio.

+ teaching me how to finally trust my own intuition more than the advice of everyone else

+ the gift of this little boy who grows in my belly, and who is already so loved in our family.

See ya later 2017. 2018… be kind.

January 3rd 2017

Being pregnant after losing a baby (or babies) is a completely different experience to those pregnancies that came before. I remember so feeling angry and so so sad after our third loss that I would never again get to enjoy a pregnancy.

I also felt incredibly jealous of anyone who was pregnant with a baby and got to experience that effortless trust that everything would work out. I had to keep to reminding myself that I *was* her for my first two pregnancies, reminding myself of how lucky I was for the experience of those two.

At that point though I was so wound up in my own anxiety that I couldn't imagine ever being able to enjoy a pregnancy again.

And now here I am.

14 weeks pregnant and doing my best to enjoy as much of it as I can. The anxiety creeps in at times. But I'm better at handling her

now. (And yes I try to think of my anxiety as this annoying imaginary friend that I just have to know how to handle in the right way).

Now when she starts to pop up I come back to the mantras I started using when we started trying again.

"I am healthy and strong and am growing a healthy baby".

Then I take a deep breath into my belly because that's the fastest way I know to calm down and stop being such a stress head.

Now, I journal her unhelpful thoughts out regularly so that she doesn't trick me into thinking they're my own.

Now, when she starts to creep in I know that voicing her crazy helps me to see that the fear is not actually my truth at all.

Pregnancy this time round IS completely different to my first two pregnancies.

For the most part with Eamon and Rory, I was blissfully naive to the experience of losing a baby. Or at least, naive to the fact that there was a chance it could happen to me and how painful it would be.

I was aware it could happen, I just foolishly thought *'it would never happen to me'*.

I'd been with my own sister when she found out her little boy had no heartbeat at 22 weeks. This was three years before I had Eamon. I'd had friends who'd had miscarriages. I knew there was a chance of course, but I guess you just tell yourself it won't happen to you.
After you've been through it though, it doesn't just feel like a chance any longer. It feels like a high possibility. It feels like someone has stacked all those statistics against you (information which really doesn't help an already anxious person in the slightest).

After three losses I resigned myself to the fact that I wouldn't get to enjoy pregnancy again. I told myself that I was okay with that, and reminded myself how lucky I was to have had two completely normal uncomplicated pregnancies.

What I didn't expect though was the experience of loss to actually make me enjoy pregnancy more, once I got a handle on the anxiety.

My eyes are fully open to the complete miracle of growing a baby now. I'm so hyper-aware of the absolute magic of it all that I'm incredibly grateful for even the bad bits (the morning sickness, my low blood pressure and the non-existent energy).

Unlike my first two pregnancies there is no internal bemoaning the process of pregnancy. There is no wishing away the 9 months or complaining that I '*Can't wait for this to be over*'. (Apologies to anyone I may have voiced this to during my first two pregnancies. I now understand your strong desire to slap me).

I've been firmly present in every moment of this pregnancy, to the point that I can actually tell you down to the day how far along I am. Each new day that clocks over feels like a huge blessing and I send out a little thank you to the universe.

Of course though, it isn't all roses. I don't think I'll be completely anxiety free until this baby is born into my hands. Actually who am I kidding, maybe not even then.

Loss has given me this other amazing gift (or curse – depending on how you want to look at it). It makes me keenly aware of how fragile life is. My mind often plays worst-case-scenarios in my head whenever my boys are away from me, especially when someone else is driving them somewhere.

I can't explain it, but my anxiety is always sky-high until I get the '*Arrived safely*' text. I say **gift** because it definitely means you can't take any of life for granted when you're so aware of how easily it can all end.

I still check every time I go to the toilet for blood. It's less of an intense, anxiety driven urge like it was during the last pregnancy. But the urge to check is definitely still there.

Waiting to feel movement has been a huge lesson in patience. I've only recently begun to feel his little kicks and rolls, far earlier than I've ever noticed it with the boys. And only because I've been desperately waiting to feel it, consciously aware of every change in my body.

Of course, now that I've felt him I want to feel him all the time for reassurance and I can get a little panicked when I haven't felt movement in a while.

Every ultrasound and doctors appointment puts my self-calming techniques to the test. My heart races, I feel sick and I literally have to chant my mantra and tell myself to breathe before each one.

Even those that are just your average, run of the mill, check blood pressure-all good-see you next month variety, send my anxiety sky-rocketing.

Now that I've written all of these anxieties on paper I feel like I've made myself out to be a total crazy person. Rather than my intention which was to tell you that I'm really enjoying this pregnancy. I really am.

I no longer take for granted the ability to create a baby and it feels like bloody magic that my body can do this.

It can, and it will. While I can't wait to meet this new little man there is not a single day of carrying him that I'm wishing away.

January 18th 2018

As we approached the 16 week mark anxiety has started to creep back in. I knew this would be a hard few weeks. Orion was 16 weeks when I delivered him and it is hard to not compare now to then. It makes no logical sense of course, but I wonder - is anyone ever logically anxious? Probably not hey?

My brain often runs away with thoughts of...'*I haven't felt him move in a while. What if he is not okay?' 'What if we've gotten this far only to have no heartbeat at the next scan?'*

I've tried all the usual tricks to get myself out of this little funk. Writing. Yoga. Talking about it. Distraction.

But it seems at this point in the pregnancy, anxiety is firmly in place as my shadow, following me around everywhere I go.

I had my first midwife appointment today at the hospital. Perhaps this too is making it all a little bit worse (I always get really anxious around appointments).

I heard his beautiful heartbeat again today, which was another moment of relief. But it was also an appointment where they did a full medical history.

I had to go through all the details of every pregnancy, followed by them tallying 6 pregnancies, *only 2 children.*

I think I've got a little case of the pregnancy blues. They caught me off guard to be honest.

I was starting to feel good. I was just getting back into teaching yoga again. And BAM.

Tears. And lots of them.

The desire to do nothing but mope about the house.

Frustration at everyone and everything.

Andrew keeps asking *'What's wrong?'* and I really don't know how to answer. Nothing. *Everything?*

I'm going to assume this is just some hormonal thing going on (I can just blame everything on hormones from here on out, can't I?)

9th February 2018

I feel profoundly sad today. For no reason that I can explain.

Perhaps it's pregnancy hormones?

Perhaps it's for everything that has happened and for all the sadness that is yet to come?

Perhaps it's for all the sad things happening in the the world right now.

I'm feeling it all.

14th February 2018

I had my 20 week ultrasound on Monday. My appointment wasn't until 1pm which meant the entire day was pretty much a write off. I spent the morning wandering the house looking for distractions. Looking for anything to take the edge off my anxiety. I literally felt like I wanted to crawl out of my own skin.

I'm sure Rory was picking up on my mood because he was weird and clingy all morning too.

I felt utterly sick walking into the scan place. My heart was beating and my stomach churning as I lay on the table. I tried to make the normal happy chit chat with the sonographer. I tried to play the role of the excited expectant Mum but it's so hard when all of my being was just waiting for the first picture, to see the flickering of his heart.

After we saw it I tried to relax, but still couldn't. My mind kept jumping to the worst case scenario.

She measured his head and had a look at his brain. My mind asked *What if there is something wrong with his brain?!"*

She looked at the four chambers of his heart. My mind jumped to *'Oh no, maybe she is taking so long because his heart isn't beating properly.'*

She looked at his spine for what felt like a decade, from every angle and position. I had to move left and right, back and forth while she tried to get the perfect image. My mind the whole time screaming at me *'What is wrong? Oh my god there is something wrong with his spine?'*

Is this a normal response to having had so many negative ultrasound experiences? I don't know. I just know that's where my brain went and it took all my restraint not to ask her every five seconds *'Is he okay? Is there something wrong?'*

At one point I did actually ask her if there was a problem because she was concentrating so hard on what she was looking at. She assured me it was just because she was trying to get the perfect picture. In the end we decided she must be fairly new because she seemed more thorough and careful than anyone I'd ever had before.

We went home assuming everything was fine, although after my experience with Orion I no longer assume that they're going to tell you if there is something wrong at the ultrasound place. They kindly leave that good news for your doctor to deliver.

I had my follow up appointment with the obstetrician today. She printed out the results and assured me it all looked normal. I sighed with relief... until she followed it up with a little comment about *'None of these tests are 100% certain, but they're pretty good.'*

I'm sure this comment was part of some standard procedure that they're meant to say for the small percentage of mothers who do have problems arise after this 20 week check. For those whose babies are born with a problem that was missed.

I get it. But I still don't want to hear it. Before Orion I barely took any notice of statistics or the potential problems. I naively assumed that my babies would always be healthy.

Back then I thought I was healthy; why wouldn't they be?

Now it's like my brain (and body) are on high alert for every potential risk. I really have to fight the urge to assume that any small percentage of risk is a sure thing for me now. It's like I default to thinking *'Yep of course, that will happen to us, because that would be my luck.'*

It's a thought pattern I have to fight daily. I have a constant soundtrack of my own positive mantras to try and drown out the doubts and fears. I wish I could say I am 100% confident in my ability to grow and birth another healthy baby, but sadly that is just not true. There are moments when I feel this as truth, but there are also many many moments where I have to work hard to control the anxiety that creeps in.

I think this is okay though. I feel the fear of potential loss daily. I am working with it and I am still here. My baby is growing perfectly and right in this moment, everything is perfect. I guess I can't ask for much more than that, can I?

29th March 2018

This pregnancy feels physically so much harder than my first two. My blood pressure is low and some days even basic tasks feel like a *real* struggle. Walking up the one flight of stairs to our front door makes me feel like I need to lie down for a nap. If I get up too fast from sitting I often see stars. Once I've done an hour or so of anything, I'm pretty much spent for the rest of the day. Even social activities tire me out super fast. It's almost like I have no energy left for anything other than growing this baby. Unfortunately though, life doesn't stop just because you're pregnant.

I often hear myself mentally saying *'Ugh this is so hard. I can't wait for this to be over'*. I then quickly try and take the thought back as fast as I can, in fear that the universe might somehow hear me and make this happen.

This is a pregnancy that I've wanted for so long. A pregnancy that I've spent so much time imagining and visualising and trying to make happen. Yet now that it's here I have to remind myself daily not to wish it away.

I feel guilty that I'm not enjoying this pregnancy as I thought I would. Shouldn't I be ecstatically happy? Shouldn't I be embracing every change? My ever-growing belly, the desire to sleep and eat all the time, the insomnia... all of these things that are signs of a healthy pregnancy?

Instead I feel heavy and awkward. Some days I feel so uncomfortable in my own body that I would crawl out of my own skin if I could.

Of course I don't always feel like this. I relish feeling our baby moving and wriggling around inside me. I love that my boys have already created their own relationship with their brother, kissing my belly hello and goodbye whenever they see me.

I feel like I'm not allowed to feel and express the negative feelings I have about this pregnancy. Like somehow, because this baby was so desperately wanted, because of the losses we've experienced before this one, that I'm somehow not allowed to have complaints about it now.

I also feel guilty when I complain because I've been on the other side too. I've been the woman who isn't pregnant but desperately wants to be and I've felt the absolute rage to hear a pregnant woman complaining about how fucking lucky she is to be carrying a healthy baby.

Which is crazy, right?

Just like everything in life, it's not black and white.

You don't have to feel the same way about everything all the time. You're allowed to change your mind (multiple times and back again). You're allowed to do everything you can to make something happen and then not enjoy the entire process once you're there.

I'm allowed to love and hate pregnancy from one minute to the next, or even at the same time.

I'm allowed to feel so so so so grateful to be carrying this healthy baby and also be really looking forward to the whole thing being over.

I'm allowed to be both amazed at my changing body and at times frustrated that it just won't do what I want it to do.

It's okay to say that I cannot wait to have this baby and at other times feel a little apprehensive about what having three children is going to be like.

It's ok to absolutely love my body when it's pregnant and at the same time feel like I really can't wait to not be pregnant anymore.

It doesn't make me a hypocrite and it doesn't make me ungrateful.

I think it just makes me human.

May 9th 2018

At 32 weeks I've finally started allowing myself to think about birth. Despite how hard I try to keep them at bay, those thoughts of *What if something goes wrong during birth?'* seem to manage to creep in every time I let myself think about it.

It's a funny kind of place to be in. In so many ways I'm incredibly connected to this little boy already. He squirms in my belly all day long. This is something that I'm so grateful for because it has helped keep the anxiety at bay.

At the same time, I often have to remind myself that there will be a new person in our family soon. Obviously I can't miss the belly now and I'm not in denial that he is here.

But I guess it's just still not a given for me that this pregnancy will be a baby, like it was with my other two. With them, as soon as I fell pregnant I began imagining myself with them in my arms. What they'd look like. How I'd feel in that first moment I laid eyes on them.

But in this pregnancy it still feels surreal to me that I will have a baby in 7 weeks. Where it was so easy to imagine my two other boys, I still struggle to imagine who this boy will be.

I guess it's normal, but sometimes I wish I could feel that quiet confidence that I had with the other two.

I am well and truly ready for this pregnancy to be over so that I can find comfort in the weight of his realness as he lays in my arms.

June 18 2018

We're getting so close now!

Part of me wishes I could hold him right now. The other part of me whispers to him *'Hold on a little bit longer.'* This is likely the last time I will ever be pregnant.

This makes both happy and terribly sad all at the same time. I love my body when I am pregnant. I love my big belly and I feel confident in how I look. Even if I am feeling more awkward than ever.

I'm often laughing at my own ridiculousness when I try and haul myself out of a chair or fit through a space I am clearly too big for.

June 19 2018

I remember vividly the last time I was in a maternity ward (the place they put you once you've had the baby, not the birthing suite).

Although the time I'm talking about was never going to end with me taking home a healthy baby.

I often have flashbacks. I can smell the hospital disinfectant. I can hear the cry of fresh babies in the rooms next door. I can feel the hustle and bustle of the hospital and remember wishing to be anywhere but there.

I remember with painful clarity exactly how I felt, even though it was over two years ago now.

I remember feeling a bit like a deer in headlights, wide-eyed, shocked and almost disbelieving that this was happening to me, to us.

I remember hours of watching mindless TV waiting for my body to start releasing a baby that it didn't really want to let go of.

I remember the moment he was born and how unlike my other births, there was no one there to catch him.

I can close my eyes and picture cradling Orion in our hands, barely able to see him for all the blankets and the tears as the midwife tenderly drew his hand out with a single finger.

I remember the midwife whispering to me as she took him away that next time would be better.

I remember feeling my body flashing hot and cold as they helped me off the toilet floor to the bed where I promptly passed out.

I remember not caring at that point if I ever woke up.

I remember feeling pissed off when I came round, only to be told I would be going to theatre after all because my body was retaining the placenta.

I remember thinking *Are you fucking kidding me? I just went through all of that and I still have to go to theatre anyway?!*

I remember feeling relieved when the physical process was over.

I remember walking from my room to the lift on the way out. I had to pass five bedroom doors, each with brand new babies and mothers inside.

I remember walking past the common room where an extended family was meeting a new baby for the first time.

I remember turning my face away and sobbing, and the look of pain on Andrew's as he watched mine.

I remember getting home to my boys and feeling overwhelmed by the feelings of sadness but also of deep gratitude (that I didn't fully understand yet.) Grateful because I now knew how much of a miracle they both were, but oh so sad because all I could think about was their brother who I had lost. And how because I had lost him all the things that they in turn had lost. All the firsts. All the love. All the craziness of what would have been three under four.

I don't remember the postpartum period or how long it took for my body to recover. I do remember they gave me a little tablet to stop my body making milk. While I'm normally someone who won't even take a panadol unless I absolutely need to, at the time I gratefully swallowed that little pill and wished they also had one to turn my mind off in the same way they could with my body.

I don't remember how I made it through those first few days or weeks, or even months. I have no recollection of what we did, or who we saw or what I said. I can however remember the excruciating pain and deep sadness that I felt and how I couldn't imagine how I would ever escape it.

I remember the extreme anxiety I felt whenever we would leave the house. Especially if we were going to see someone for the first time since we'd lost Orion. It's funny how time in my head is now divided into "before" and "after."

I'll carry these memories with me always. Though despite the pain of them I've now come to a place where I wouldn't choose to skip any of them even if I could. These are my only experiences *of him* and I am grateful for them.

I remember feeling at the time that I wasn't strong enough to bear the weight of all of it.

But I am.

We are.

This still amazes me. We are so much stronger than we even know and it takes the shittiest of experiences to show us.

The last few weeks of this pregnancy I've felt lighter. (Not physically obviously – because I'm heavier than I've ever been and totally committed to #pregnantcarblife)

But emotionally… mentally… spiritually – I feel lighter. A little more like my 'before' self, but still a very changed version of me.

Don't get me wrong, I am still feeling scared and anxious at times – after all he is not yet in my arms.

But mostly I feel that excitement and joy about life again. Something I hadn't really even realised I was missing.

So here's to happy endings… that are really just new beginnings after all.

July 5th 2018

He's here, he's perfect and parts of me still can't completely believe it.

Despite having thought about him and dreamed of him for the better part of two years it feels surreal to finally have him in my arms.

The last two years now feel hazy. Like I know I lived it but I'm not 100% sure how I survived it. Almost like I have to ask myself *Did that really happen?*

How did I even get through all that?

I expected to break down emotionally when I gave birth. Surprisingly I didn't. Of course it was the emotional roller coaster that birth usually is, but that moment where I picked him up and brought him to my chest was the same happy, crazy, amazing moment that it was with Eamon and Rory.

I was just in awe of this little person who felt like he came from no where was now in my arms. (Not literally of course, I bloody well FELT where he came from).

It wasn't until after, that my emotions of the three who came before him came rushing in to remind me exactly how miraculous this moment really was.

Out of the blue the other night Eamon asked me how many babies did I have that weren't born. On day four no less – notoriously known as one of the most emotional days postpartum.

I was feeding Luca at the time and just looked down at him and burst into tears.

He knew about Orion, but I'd never directly spoken about our other two losses.

He knew of course. Both boys have this strange psychic ability to know when I'm pregnant. Just days after I would have been pregnant with Luca, Rory put his hand on my belly and said *'Baby'* and Eamon randomly came out with a statement like *'Mum I just had this thought that you had a baby in your belly'* laughed and then walked off.

I didn't yet know of course. It was literally only days after he was conceived and no pregnancy test in the world would show that up.

But I also knew, you know?

I hadn't outwardly spoken to Eamon about the two losses after Orion but I have no doubt he felt them. I also know from Andrew that he had at one point asked *'When will Mummy stop being sad and sick all the time?'*

The thought of him feeling this way broke my heart.

So while it was strange for him to be asking about these babies now, I guess it was probably a long overdue conversation.

'What do you mean?' I asked first (because sometimes I interpret his questions wrong and give him too much information.)

'Like how many babies did you have before Luca that weren't born like Rory and I?'

Yep, no misinterpreting that.

'Three' I croaked trying to hold back tears.

Rory thought about this for a while and piped in with *'But where are they now?'*

At that point the tears fell.

Where are they? I don't know how to answer that?

No where?

Everywhere?

With me always.

Mum jumped in to answer them while I cried hot happy sad tears onto the head of my rainbow baby.

To be honest I've never really connected with the whole 'rainbow baby' concept. I understand the idea, but for me losing babies doesn't just make the baby born after loss extra special, it makes those born *at all* total bloody miracles.

I feel like I appreciate my boys so much more because of my losses and with Luca I just feel so so lucky that I get to experience all of his baby stages with lucid awareness of how magic it all is.

So despite the fact that day 2 and 3 postpartum were as incredibly hard as they usually are. It hurt to sit, my nipples were on fire from his dodgy latch, I hadn't slept in days and he wanted to feed round the clock because my milk hadn't come in yet.

I was also incredibly aware of how amazing these hard bits are too and I felt grateful for having them to experience at all. (And yes I can feel gratitude and still also grumble *'Go the fuck to sleep'* under my breath in the dark of the night).

It's 4am as I type this. Luca is asleep on my chest after sleeping for four hours, which after days of zero sleep feels like all I need. He is 6 days old today.

I feel grateful and tired. Delighted in his every movement, yet also mildly frustrated when he cries for yet another feed. I am extended beyond what even feels possible when three little people need me for something all at once and yet also completely content with it all.

It's all the feelings. All at once. One after the other.

It's everything.

PART TWO - YOUR STORIES

Bec Kenny

I can't even tell you how much of a support Bec has been to me over the past two years. After each loss she reached out to share her story with me. Each time only delivering just the right amount of information for me to handle. I didn't know the full extent of her losses until after my third. In many ways I'm glad she shielded me somewhat from this information until I was ready to face the full truth of what some women go through to create their family. I think I may have given up after Orion if I'd known I would have to go through two more losses before I carried another healthy baby. I can't even imagine how Bec has managed to pick herself back up and go on after each of her losses. I am in awe of how she manages to still have such a positive and happy approach to life despite all of the challenges she's faced.

Bec's story is one of amazing strength, resilience and profound love for her babies. She has taught me so much, but most importantly she showed me the importance of holding onto hope even through the most negative of times. She taught me to water the flowers, not the weeds and I will be forever grateful to her for that.

I am a mother of 4 beautiful healthy kids, but that is not the end of my story. My last baby born was my 14th pregnancy. I love my big family and I hope my story shows you that you should never let anything get in the way of your dreams.

I had a termination of pregnancy at 23 years old and the whole time I was afraid that I would never fall pregnant again. I was worried I wouldn't be able to have kids because I had ended that pregnancy and there would be complications. I had also previously been told that I had a good chance of infertility given my cycles, so it was a huge concern. But at the time I was basically single, wasn't in a serious relationship and I was strongly encouraged to choose this option.

In 2005 I met the love of my life, we got engaged and started our family pretty much straight away.

Our first daughter was born in 2006 after an extremely traumatic birth. She had severe shoulder dystocia and I experienced severe haemorrhaging. I had to give my consent to have a hysterectomy if they could not stop the bleeding. As I said goodbye to my newborn daughter and fiancé, the likely outcome did not look positive. Luckily the Doctors and two blood transfusions saved my life.

It was not an easy road to recovery. It was 16 weeks before I could walk properly again and I was strongly urged to not to try having a natural birth again, only caesareans.

We were married in 2007 and I had a miscarriage at 8 weeks.

In 2008 I delivered my first son by Caesarian.

In 2010 I miscarried two babies at 7 weeks.

In 2011 our second daughter was born by Caesarian.

In 2012 I had another miscarriage at 8 weeks.

In 2013 I had four miscarriages all at the 8 week mark.

In January of 2014 I delivered our baby boy Huey at 21 weeks. He was born sleeping.

My pregnancy with Huey was going well, all my scans were normal. I had my check up at 20 weeks, a week before scan. My midwife wasn't confident she found the heartbeat, but I had a scan a couple of days later so didn't think much of it. I still felt movements so I was confident that all was well.

My 20 week scan was scheduled for 9am. I was on my own as husband wasn't able to make it.

The sonographer said *'I will be back soon, I just need to check something'*. I knew what we were seeing wasn't normal. After all I'd been here many times before. I knew what he was going to say.

He eventually came back in and said *'I'm really sorry, your baby has no heartbeat'*.

My first thought was *'Why? Why does he not have a heartbeat, can you see why?'* We found out later that had Huey actually passed away 4 weeks earlier and I'd had no idea. There was a slight indication that the cord slowly came away forming a blood clot. It was slow and probably why I'd still felt him moving.

The sonographer was a wonderful man. He organised for me to be able to just to walk out of the clinic without paying or doing any paperwork, and made sure I was okay. I was in shock at the time. I rang my husband and my Mum and just cried. Feeling incredibly lost I also rang my obstetrician and went in to see her.

It was really challenging walking into a clinic with so many pregnant women after having just found out I'd lost my baby. They moved me into a private office where I was alone waiting for the OB to arrive. In that moment I found my rational thinking and realised that I needed to get this baby out. I knew that the chance of me becoming seriously ill could be very real. I knew I needed to move focus on the children I do have, so I needed to get back to being healthy.

My obstetrician rang the hospital and they had a spare room so it was booked for me immediately. I pushed to have the process done as soon as possible. My OB praised my rational thinking given the circumstances. I have a good relationship with her although she wasn't there at Huey's birth.

I went home and organised a babysitter for our kids and got myself organised. We returned to hospital at around 3pm and they started the process of what was to be a very long night. The medication they gave me was not working so I requested a caesarean but they said it was too dangerous as baby was too low.

They increased my medication and I ended up having an epidural though it didn't work as I was already too far along.

At 9 am I delivered Huey NATURALLY. Yes he was stillborn but I delivered him. Being able to have another natural birth, which I never thought I would do, was an amazing experience. I stayed in hospital for 2 days. The only regret I have is not showing Huey to the other children because I was so self-absorbed at the time. I thought I was doing the right thing but I denied them the chance to see their brother. I realised once I got home that I'd made a mistake. It would have helped them heal and to answer all their questions. They were a part of this journey too and I believe it would have created some closure for them.

Afterwards the placenta was manually removed. This was excruciatingly painful. Ten times worse than birth. The registered OB didn't get it all the first time and had to try again. I felt violated at the time, as I felt it was being done against my will or consent and I filed a complaint afterwards.

After Huey was born they put a butterfly sticker on my door as code to let others know to keep the door shut. They never asked if I wanted it opened. No one (staff) really talked to me. I assume they thought I needed space and time, but for me I felt isolated and like I had done something wrong.

I wanted the door open. I wanted to see people. I'd just had a baby like everyone else. My milk was coming in like everyone else. My body was hurting like everyone else. Why was I being treated so differently? I understand that if this was my first, it may have been different, but it was the fact no one even asked me. No one bothered to ask the simple little things like whether I would like the door left open or a cup of tea when the cart came round in the morning.

I did make the hospital aware of it afterwards, hoping I could prevent other mothers feeling the same way. There were also conflicting information about what would happen to Huey's remains. I was confused by the system and I was very lucky that Huey was still there when I changed my mind and decided to have him cremated so that I could bring him home.

The worst part about this whole experience were the things no one talks about. The nightmares I experienced were unbearable. I had visions of my youngest getting eaten by a toy crocodile, which sounds crazy, but it felt so real. Five days later I ended up with a severe kidney and bladder infection. I went to the doctor who gave me antibiotics, but it turned out I was allergic to them.

I remember it was a 40 degree day and I couldn't get warm, then my heart was racing and my throat started to close over. I rang my husband to come home straight away and we went straight back to hospital. It took a few weeks to recover physically from this whole ordeal.

Despite our short time together with Huey he taught me so much about myself. I am forever grateful for that. Although his physical life may have ended I know his soul is alive and well.

I never feared having more children after all of my losses as I was grateful for every single one of them. **I knew if I could live through them, I could live through anything** and I became stronger within myself. At the end of 2014 I delivered our baby daughter by caesarian.

When I reflect on all of our babies I think that my thoughts became very toxic when I was pregnant with Huey. I was taking on board a lot of negative opinions and energies of other people. I was so worried what others would think of me having a 4th child. I look back and I do wonder whether this was some of the reason that my pregnancy ended? I do not blame myself but I have strongly learnt from this and that in itself was a major lesson Huey taught me. I learnt to spend my time concentrating on the flowers in my garden and not on the weeds.

I could spend a lot of time grieving over my losses, but I don't. I am grateful for the experiences they have brought me. Even though their lives were so short, I was grateful I fell pregnant in the first place.

I'm grateful to carry a living being inside of me; this is denied to so many! I am grateful for the deliveries and so amazed at the ability of my body to heal itself. I am also grateful that I have helped these little souls complete a part of their journey.

No one can take away the feeling of carrying a child, of being a mother, of all the changes my body has been through and the emotions these losses have made me feel.

I do get stuck on the question *"How many kids do you have?"* though. Most of the time I say 4 but I know I have 5 and that's all that matters to me .

Never lose focus on your dreams and what is right for you. This is your life, your journey and your story.

Lisa De Hosson

Lisa and I have been in contact many times since I lost Orion. Her friendship is yet another example of how amazing the internet can be in drawing two people, who otherwise would have never met, together. Right from the start she openly shared her pain over losing her daughter Georgie and I felt safe to share the rawness of my feelings in the early days with her. Her story is a beautiful example of the strength of a Mother's intuition and the love she will always hold for Georgie.

Her.

Georgie Dawn de Hosson – 28/05/2015

We found out we were pregnant a few minutes before midnight on December 31, 2014. I wanted to do the test before the year clicked over so I could start it on a high. Little did I know at that time that 2015 would also bring me the lowest low I'd ever had. But like her name suggests; the sun will rise again every day and with that there is always hope.

My initial blood tests returned a very high Beta HCG reading. I work for my GP so he rang me laughing, suggesting I might be carrying twins. I was sent for an early dating scan at 6 weeks and the sonographer said *'There is no heartbeat but I can see one sac'*. My heart jumped until I remembered at that young age the heart hasn't started to beat yet. After a few more weeks of blood tests it was assumed that a second baby may not have developed as far as Georgie had and my levels started to settle.

The rest of the pregnancy was uneventful until around 20 weeks when my sciatic nerve started to render me useless. At 23 weeks I had a remedial massage, and the massage therapist kept talking to me about how she is psychic and can predict things happening to people but she isn't sure how people will respond. Thinking back to those words gives me goosebumps now.

By 24 weeks we were getting wardrobes installed in bub's room and planning new carpet. We weren't finding out the gender so we were beginning to get very excited. We went for dinner on the Friday night with our 22 month old daughter. I remember feeling very pregnant all of a sudden and as we walked back to the car in the rain, I felt so happy with how everything was going. I went to bed that night truly happy. It was the last time in my life that I would ever feel that happy.

On the Saturday morning I went for a massage at a day spa. The young therapist continually talked about Eurovision but I couldn't concentrate as I had a niggling thought that I couldn't remember when I had last felt Georgie move. That afternoon I went to the physio to get some acupuncture and more treatment on my sciatic nerve. By that stage I felt a little more concerned but brushed it off as I'd had such a busy morning.

By Saturday night I felt….different. As if I knew, but didn't want to admit it yet. There was no sickness, no pain, no bleeding….nothing. My husband made me a spicy curry and we went to bed early. I did not sleep a wink.

On Sunday morning I rang the hospital to get the old *'Have a cold drink and lay on your left side'* lecture. My intuition was screaming at me, but I wasn't brave enough at that stage to enter the world of a bereaved mother, so I did as I was told. I laid on our bed while my husband painted around me. I was in the sun listening to my Calmbirth tracks, willing to feel any movement. Even though the sun was directly on me, I've never felt so cold.

I phone my GP and he met me at work to listen for the heartbeat. He suggested we go to the hospital and get checked out.

My husband was painting our room when I got home and said he knew as soon I walked in. My sister took our daughter to their place and we left for the hospital, taking the longest way by accident. Or perhaps not.

The midwives put me into the room I'd had my daughter in not quite two years before. The room where as a first time mother I presented to hospital fully dilated and pushing. The room where previously I'd had the most beautiful birth. The room that saw the start of our family. Now I was hooked up to a CTG machine listening to my racing heartbeat and the well-meaning midwives saying that bub must be hiding or that *'Ooh, was that it?'* I really wished they didn't say those things. I hated the sound of my heartbeat for a long long time after that.

Finally my obstetrician was called and he walked in and said it didn't sound good did it? He called for an ultrasound machine and there she was, lying so still, so perfect. My poor husband broke. I was in shock, I remember wondering what the football score was in the background while staring at the image of my baby on the screen.

Next came all the questions.

When to induce *(induce!?)*
What will happen?

We made the phone calls to parents that we really didn't want to make. As if saying those words would make it true.

We decided that we would induce on the Wednesday. My obstetrician let us choose when, and let us know we could change our minds at any time. Nothing would happen until we were induced. We are so glad we took those extra three days. It meant we could go home late that Sunday night and let what happened sink in. We were able to gather the support we needed and prepare for the birth and what lay ahead.

Coming home that night was so hard. My parents and sister were here with our daughter and our GP was here waiting for us too. After working with him for so long, I knew he was used to attending scenes like this and administering something to help people calm down or sleep, but I was shocked to find I wasn't teary in the slightest. I had to be strong for my daughter, and my family.

During the few days at home we had concrete trucks coming to pour slabs, florists coming with bunch after bunch, and the heartbreak of having to think of funerals and burials. I ended up having a big breakdown in Target as I realised there weren't any nappies that were going to fit her, or clothes. We ended up in Pumpkin Patch trying to buy their teddy bear clothes except they only had leggings with unicorns on them and the sales girl was young and really unsympathetic to our situation. Thankfully my mother-in-law made a gown and it was absolutely perfect. The midwives took care of the nappy.

By the time the morning of my induction came around we had made so much peace with what had happened. We realised our sadness came from mourning the future that we were never promised with our child, or with anyone for that matter, and that we had to be grateful for the blessings we had received from this experience. As we drove over the mountain overlooking the beach, the sun was rising and it was such a beautiful view. We had said that if the baby was born as the sun rose it was going to be a girl, and Dawn would be her middle name. This also stemmed from the saying that my Dad lives by; *"The sun will rise everyday and we will keep on going."*

The first Misoprostol tablet was inserted at 7:50am that morning, Wednesday May 27. We were told that it can take anywhere from 24-48 hours for things to start happening and to sit tight. I would be having a tablet inserted every 4 hours after that. My ob was quite somber and I berated him, telling him that if he wanted to be a part of this birth he had better wear a happy face as we were still having our second baby!

I decided to pop my Calmbirth tracks on and start visualising to see if I could get things going a bit quicker. We ate and rested all day and started watching the State of Origin that night. I thought I could feel things changing and my cervix was starting to efface by that afternoon. My OB came to visit and told us to prepare for a few days of waiting. He said we could have a tablet at 7pm, then 11pm and then leave overnight until the next morning so that I could rest.

All during the night I could hear a woman in labour. I kept waiting for that moment where she would push and I'd hear a baby cry. I so desperately wanted to hear a baby cry. She was eventually taken to theatre and I got some sleep.

At 5am that morning the midwife came in and inserted another tablet. She was quite surprised and she said *'I think you're going to have your baby today'* which was nice to hear, as I hadn't felt anything else change and had been asleep with no tablet for the last six hours.

By 7am breakfast came and it was eggs. I hate eggs and the smell of them made me irrationally angry. Gav was wondering why I was like this. My OB came in just after 7am on his way to theatre and said I would be here for awhile yet. I was listening but didn't have much to say. He left and I paced the room ranting about the smell of the breakfast, when suddenly I got the urge to go to the toilet, like when you have food poisoning. I remembered the midwives telling me to buzz and not go to the toilet so I jumped on the bed. I pushed the buzzer once and then the urge to push was so overwhelming that I pushed the buzzer again whilst trying to rip my pants off. Three midwives burst into the room and before they could get their gloves on out came my baby en caul (born in the sac.) Someone ran to the hallway to yell for my OB who came running back. He was perplexed as to what he just felt in the exam, then seeing the sac on the table.

It looked beautiful, a full balloon of water, a healthy level no doubt. He cut the sac open and lifted our baby out for me to pull up on to me. It felt like any other birth, perfect.

My warm baby cuddled up on my chest. I was saying to my husband 'What did we have?' and he was saying 'I think we have another girl'. Of course we did. It was too good to be true. Another beautiful daughter.

I remember noticing that the sun was just starting to shoot rays across the room through the slatted blinds. It was 7:47am, less than twenty minutes of labour and our 1lb 1oz 35cm baby girl Georgie Dawn was here.

One thing I remember so vividly is my OB crying when he lifted her out of her sac. He looked her over and was saying 'She's perfect'. There was nothing physically wrong, the placenta and cord were both fine. Everything was as it should be. I ended up having ten vials of blood taken and her placenta sent away to pathology and all of the results were normal. It was a completely unexplained stillbirth.

After the birth, we spent a whole day with her creating many wonderful memories before we handed her over to the funeral director. A midwife let us walk her through the hospital in an open basket for everyone to see. Georgie's final walk was with her parents so proud and devastated. My husband said it was the proudest he had felt.

The next part was truly the worst moment of my life, watching my baby drive off and knowing I will never see her again. I still don't know how I got through that moment. I turned around and the sky looked so magnificent that I took a photo. **It was like I knew then that if I could get through that moment I could get through anything.**

As for healing, that was strange. The bleeding had ceased by two weeks and my milk never came in after my OB gave me a tiny tablet that knocks the supply off. I wanted the recovery to be longer, almost as if I wanted to hold on to the whole experience.

The next few weeks seemed to pass in a blur. I remember having a few cries here and there, mainly in the shower at night. I couldn't shower alone so my husband had to sit with me while I showered. Mainly I just felt numb. We had a lot of family and friends really avoid us during this time and that seemed to make all the hurt so much worse. We not only lost our daughter but most of our friends and surprisingly, a lot of family too. This is a major source of hurt but now we mostly look at it as a blessing. Our daughter culled all the people from our lives that didn't want to be there for us at our worst and now don't deserve to be with us at our best. We are now surrounded by those who we can count on and it's nice to know those relationships have been bolstered by our experience.

Georgie was cremated and we picked her up on a freezing yet sunny Friday afternoon. We took her for a drive and then decided we should celebrate her coming home like we would normally do with a newborn baby, albeit a bit differently. So eleven days after our last family dinner we went out again with her. She proudly sat on our table and we had champagne to toast her coming home to us. It was such a memorable night. The next morning was her service, at a seaside heritage listed area where we were married four years before. We wanted it to be as the sun rose and asked our closest family to join us. We were saddened when some chose their holiday over supporting us. It left my husband shattered and is something we still struggle to forgive. I'm sure he was drawing on the strength of our daughter to get him through. As the sun rose over the sea we played some especially chosen songs and everyone wrote a message on a balloon to release, including our eldest daughter. It was perfect.

Then.

We went to see our OB two weeks after she was born. He was so fantastic the entire time. He asked us how we felt about future children. We were of course nervous, but he reassured us that the fact Georgie's death was unexplained meant that there was no foreseeable risk or problem to monitor with the next pregnancy (besides increased anxiety.) He advised us to at least wait until Georgie's due date before we tried again and that would also take us past her first birthday. He warned us that these first milestones would be hard and they were.

At first I wanted a baby straight away. I had all of this newborn energy with no newborn to channel it into. I felt cheated. Every time I heard someone announce a pregnancy I would get so angry. I was angry that people were so carefree announcing their pregnancies, as if nothing was going to happen to them. I was anxious for them, and would continue to be until baby was born and a healthy birth announcement was made. Not long afterwards our friends suffered a traumatic miscarriage and it threw me to dark depths I had just crawled out of.

For Georgie's due date we escaped down to our favourite place on the south coast of NSW. We wanted to be away from everyone and everything. It ended up being the most beautiful weekend and something we have turned into an annual event.

Once her due date passed I told her to send us a baby when we were ready. Three weeks later I woke up with a wet top, colostrum leaking through overnight. I was still 4-5 days away from my period and only lasted a few days before I was due to take a pregnancy test which, unsurprisingly, was positive. The first twelve weeks I was okay, as there was no movement I had to keep track of. I had all of my tests and everything was fine, I felt tiredness and nausea but after my previous two pregnancies these seemed to bother me less.

Our twelve week scan was fine and we embarked on a heavily monitored pregnancy.

I had a key word that I took from my Calmbirth class that I did during my first pregnancy – *surrender*. That has helped me through all of my pregnancies, labours, births and most significantly, all the stuff that comes after.

When I felt the anxiety starting to build I repeatedly had to tell myself to surrender to it all. That I have no control over anything besides what I am letting myself feel, and that what will be, will be.

It sounds easy enough written on paper but the entire pregnancy was plagued by insomnia, moments of panic, despair, guilt and a myriad of other feelings. I was worried I wouldn't be able to connect with this baby, that loving this baby would push Georgie further out of the picture. For I still have to parent her, for eternity. She is my second daughter and I am responsible for keeping her memory at the forefront of our lives.

Amongst all of this was our first Christmas without Georgie. I was only three months pregnant so no-one really knew at this stage except for my closest family and friends. We wanted to keep it that way for as long as possible. When it came time to decorate the house for Christmas, I had a panic attack. I felt the overwhelming burden of trying to be excited and happy for our two year old but the pain and aching loss made me feel so guilty about it. Even now I find with a happy occasion comes a debilitating bout of guilt that I've learnt to tread lightly through instead of trying to ignore it.

That first Christmas I crashed my car twice in one week and quickly learnt that ignoring those feelings doesn't work. We announced our pregnancy to the rest of the family on Christmas morning which was mostly met with happiness. There were still some who were unhappy with how we'd handled the announcement. They didn't seem to understand that the reason we'd been cold and distant since our daughter's funeral was because we felt hurt and unsupported by them back then.

We opted to find out the gender at our 19 week scan. We felt bad we didn't know Georgie's gender and I wondered how (as someone who loves to be organised) I had gotten through all the scans without wanting to know. In hindsight though it was like I wasn't meant to know, that by not knowing I couldn't get completely attached to the idea of Georgie being my living baby girl.

Our 'rainbow baby' (a term that makes me cranky for some reason, and that's just my opinion) was a girl. She gave me the smoothest pregnancy of the three, as if she'd been told to treat me gently. Of course I worried about how I would manage a toddler and newborn on top of what we had been through. I also worried how I would manage all the well-wishers who suddenly thought they could come out of the woodwork and be happy for us again, like we would be cured by this new baby. I had so many people tell me before I fell pregnant that I should hurry up and have another baby, as if it would make the pain go away, but I felt like it was more so they didn't have to keep having these awkward conversations. No-one tells a widow to hurry up and re-marry, do they?!

By Georgie's first birthday I was 36 weeks pregnant. Her first birthday was a really happy time. That morning we went to the place where we'd held her funeral and had breakfast there as the sun rose. Again, it was so perfect. I often feel when she is with me and I knew she was there that morning. When we came home my family helped us celebrate with a little party and cake which thrilled our eldest daughter. She is so proud and protective of Georgie and always says that she has two sisters when people ask, and that Georgie is in heaven.

At 39 weeks + 6 days I was 4cm dilated in my OB's office without feeling a thing. I went off to hospital to have my waters broken and 2 hours later Daisy arrived. She was put on my chest blue and not breathing. As I'd endured another rapid birth, she'd made her descent down the birth canal so quickly that I went from 5cm and feeling the urge to push to dilating as she was descending, which meant I skipped transition but the pushing part was very painful.

Because of her quick descent alarm bells started ringing because her heart rate had dropped to 50 beats per minute instead of being above 120-130bpm. We were terrified. I remember looking at my husband and thinking that we could not go through this again. I had to get her out and in three mighty pushes she was here. I lifted her on to me and the nurses quickly took her to suction out the fluid that is usually squeezed out during their time coming through the birth canal. At 8lb 1oz 54cm, my little chubby bub was completely fine and she came back and latched on to feed for well over an hour.

Now.

Now I tell people that time does not heal all wounds and can we please all stop using clichés! I know people mean well, but my tolerance since we lost Georgie for clichés has been obliterated. Time only helps you to adjust and it's continual, it will never end. I will forever wonder what she would have sounded like, looked like and smelled like at every single stage. Daisy was born with an identical mouth and for weeks I cried and kissed it non stop, never wanting it to change as it looked so much like Georgie's. I remember for weeks after Georgie was born I couldn't wash Grace's hands in the bath because they had similar fingers and holding them made me want to be sick.

But now my little family is complete and I have never felt more happy or content in all of my life. A lot of people don't understand how we can say that, but Georgie's state of being was always going to be that way, and how could we wish that she had never happened? At first I felt bad for Daisy, thinking that if Georgie had lived she wouldn't be here, but I like to think three girls were always in my fate somehow.

I'm not sure how other peoples relationships fare when it comes to their experiences but even after thirteen years and three daughters together, I didn't think it would be possible for my husband and I to be any closer. Every now and then we marvel at our journey together. We remember being surprised by the closeness we experienced after we lost Georgie, almost like an intense passion. We felt a little awkward about it before being told by our OB that he had seen it before and that it most definitely wasn't unusual.

One thing I would like others to know and something I wished I had known, was to not subscribe to the 'stages of grieving'. You do not progress through them systematically nor do they all necessarily come at all. I was unhelpfully told that I would crash and burn six weeks afterwards, so naturally I spent that time counting down my apparent demise, to find that not only did it not come, but that I needed to be more wary of taking on too much of what other people said.

I was also asked if I felt guilty for what happened, like I had had any control over it. That sat awfully heavy on my shoulders. I guess some women do for their own reasons, but I truly didn't. My belief was that Georgie knew her fate and still chose our family to be born into so that she would be loved and remembered forever. Not that I had or hadn't done something to cause what happened, or that my body had failed me. My body has given me a beautiful daughter, and two others as well.

I'm not sure what the hardest part of going forward is going to be. I think now I have learnt not to think about it, to just let it happen. Just the other day we drove past a building that had doors which looked like a morgue and immediately after there was a funeral home sign and I completely lost it. I never know when that is going to happen and I know now to just surrender to the times I need to lay low and grieve for her instead of trying to push on. My life has been so blessed and I can only be grateful for everything she has given us.

Melissa Frost

One of the striking things that I remember when Melissa first reached out to me after I lost Orion was how she mentioned that her loss 'wasn't as bad' as mine because she was 'only' 7 weeks pregnant at the time. I'm not sure where we get this idea from, but it's one that I've heard echoed many times since from other women who shared their stories of miscarriage with me. We don't mourn a person any less or more because of their age and a baby who dies before they're born isn't any different. They are still a real baby to us. We know them already. We love them already. I wanted to share Melissa's story for this very reason. I want it to be written down and recognised. Don't diminish your loss or your pain around losing your baby however many weeks they are. Your loss is important. They are important. Your feelings are important.

I was 7 weeks pregnant when I woke up in the morning and noticed some spotting. I immediately felt that something was very, very wrong. (It probably didn't help that this was my first pregnancy, I went into panic mode.)

I called a co-worker (who is really like a mother to me). She said that it might be nothing, but I should call our boss and have the day off work just to be sure. I wasn't able to get in for a scan immediately - I had to wait until 2.30 that afternoon. The scan showed that everything was fine so I reassured myself that it was nothing and it was just me being paranoid. I then attended my personal training session for the week (just doing arm exercises), because the person conducting the scan had advised me that everything was normal. When I got home from training, I found that the bleeding had become heavier and this continued throughout the night.

Given that it was the end of the school year and I'm a teacher, it had been a big deal taking a day off work the previous day. I didn't believe I could ask for another day off so I went to work, even though the bleeding continued. By first break, I was laying down on my desk because of the terrible cramps. I had heavy bleeding, but knew that the chances of finding another relief staff member were slim, so I stuck it out until the end of the day.

The heavy bleeding and cramps continued again during the night. My husband was away and I didn't want to worry him, so I tried to tell myself that everything was fine.

The next day, my husband arrived home. I told him what had happened the previous day and he thought we should go to the hospital. I didn't want to go, because I thought it was better not knowing than finding out I'd lost the baby. I also didn't want the Doctors to think I was being dramatic, if it was considered normal. He eventually convinced me to go.

When we arrived at emergency, I had to tell the staff member at the front desk what was happening, then I had to repeat this to a triage nurse, then I was ushered in to see a Doctor (where I had to repeat my story again). The Doctor on duty performed an internal examination and believed my cervix was closed (which she thought was a positive sign).

She said that being a weekend, there wasn't much anyone could do and it probably wouldn't be worth the trip to Toowoomba. I was advised to make an appointment with my Doctor on the Monday and have another scan.

The bleeding continued over the weekend and on Monday I had another scan, where we were advised that I'd had a complete miscarriage (there was no foetus present).

We initially only told a couple of people that we are close with. We didn't want to tell our parents. We didn't want it to be a drama, and partly because we didn't want people to feel sorry for us. I also told my co-worker that I'd called the morning the miscarriage started

Everyone we did tell were extremely caring and supportive, offering anything they could do to help *(though of course there wasn't, I just wanted to be left alone to feel shitty!)*

About a month later, I told my mother in law. She was extremely supportive and let me cry as much as I wanted. It seemed to really set in about a month after the miscarriage. Surprisingly, I didn't feel that she pitied our situation, she just wanted to care for both of us.

I wish that I could have allowed myself to be honest with more people (I HATE feeling vulnerable). I often just try to brush it off saying, *'It is what it is'* and by thinking about how lucky I was to have my husband. I wish I could have said how I really felt - *'I'm really struggling with this and I'm scared we'll never have children'.*

I didn't take any time off work - report cards were due and I felt that I needed to keep up appearances. (Parents were already asking questions about my one day off). It was the biggest mistake, because my body started to fight against me.

While I was in denial about the miscarriage, I pushed myself to be normal by not having any time off work, continuing working out etc. Although my body had healed from the miscarriage, other things started to go wrong. My belly button piercing that I'd had since I was 16 got badly infected. I then had a UTI (which I had never had before). I was given antibiotics to treat that, but I had an allergic reaction to them, so I ended up with a terrible skin rash all over my body.

Initially, we wanted to be strong for each other, so didn't say *'This is absolutely crap, I'm devastated'.* But in the days following, we got better at showing small parts of our hurt to each other. I believe it helped us to show each other a more vulnerable side of ourselves, not just the shiny, happy side.

My husband was mostly my concerned with my wellbeing through the loss. He really started to notice how much I push myself and how much extra stress I take on. He was more open about his desire to have a family and his disappointment/sadness around the miscarriage.

We occasionally talk about our loss - whether that baby is watching over our new baby, or whether the baby returned to us as our little boy.

The most helpful thing I did was attending an appointment with an alternative healer (specialising in crystal healing, auras etc). It was so wonderful speaking to someone outside of the situation to say all of the things I felt I couldn't say. To say that I was worried my body had done this (because of the amount I stress), or that I felt I had disappointed my husband and family, or that I was terrified that I'd never be able to have a family.

The most helpful things people did for us was asking about the miscarriage. I feel like there is so much unsaid about miscarriage. I often feel like I can't start a conversation about it without people feeling sorry for us and pitying the situation. I feel like I can't spread awareness, because people will automatically feel sorry for me personally, instead of realising that miscarriage is so much more common than they realise.

It's been just over a year since we lost our baby. I'm coping well now though there are still some days where I feel sadness about the situation or wonder what could have been. But I'm extremely grateful for where I am now in life.

We found out I was pregnant again two months after our miscarriage. Our little boy is now 4 months old. At first, I was extremely cautious about the pregnancy - trying to keep stress low and only doing gentle exercise. After 7 weeks, I was a little less worried. After 13 weeks, I felt a little safer, and then again at 20 weeks. I didn't feel relieved until we held our little boy though. I was petrified of him being stillborn.

The hardest thing for me now is trying not to stress about the fragility of life. Even though our little boy is healthy, I check him constantly because I'm worried about SIDS. I'm sure when he's at school I'll be constantly worried that he could be involved in an accident while there. Having said that, I've gotten better from when he was born (I no longer have a need to check his breathing every ten minutes).

I wish I knew how common miscarriage was when I had one. Even though they tell you the statistics, it really feels like you're the only one. It's only when you start talking with others that they tell you their stories.

Rhyannon Preston

I relate to the devastation in Rhyannon's words especially when she writes about the heartache of being treated for miscarriage in the maternity ward and of not knowing how she'll ever get out of the darkness after losing two babies in a row. I've definitely been there. I remember wandering the house thinking 'How will I ever feel better?!'

Yet here we both are. Not just because our stories involved future babies, although that is certainly a part of both our stories. But because we made it through the darkness. I hope this story helps to show you that you will too.

I have never really sat down and put my story together. I look back and can't believe I made it through that time. It feels therapeutic to share my story.

Back in 2013 my husband and I went on the most amazing trip to Paris, Morocco and Turkey. This was our last 'hoorah' before we started trying for a baby.

It only took three months to fall pregnant - however it felt like years as I did so much with my diet, acupuncture and finances to prepare for this.

I knew I was pregnant before I even took the test at the crack of dawn one morning. I ran in to share with my husband and everything was bliss. We shortly shared the news with our families.

Over the next two weeks I experienced cramping every day but put this down to my body adjusting to the pregnancy. But I couldn't hide this feeling of dread I felt in the pit of my stomach and at the end of the day when my world became quieter. I found myself crying every night. The nights my husband were away were worse (he's FIFO). But I just put these feelings down to hormones.

At the six week scan there wasn't much to see and the ultrasound technician wouldn't tell me anything except for *'Go see your doctor'* and *'It's just early days.'*

I felt so fearful but tried so hard to remain positive. The light daily cramping continued. I felt that if I lied to myself and remained positive, the worst wouldn't be true. I saw my doctor and she encouraged me to wait 10 days before having another scan as she again told me *'It was early days.'*

The next part was torturous. Every day was so long and my emotions were up and down like a yoyo. I think I knew in my gut what was happening but I didn't want to admit it. My husband had to return back out to work and I desperately tried to remain positive.

On a Tuesday night, not long after midnight I woke and felt wet. I went to the toilet. When I wee at night I do it in the dark with my eyes closed, but something this time told me to turn the light on.

And there it was. So much blood.

I ran and phoned mum and couldn't even say anything. She just knew. Later she told me she knew in her gut weeks out what was happening, and even knew it would be that night.

I sobbed on the floor not knowing what to do. Should I call my husband and wake him? But he needed to sleep for his massive shift at work. There was nothing he could do. I didn't want to worry him.

Mum arrived within minutes, cleaned me up, made me a cup of tea and sat with my in front of TV. I felt numb and just cried. I think I might have fallen asleep.

I rang my husband early in the morning. He was shattered and demanded to jump on a plane and come home early. I told him not to worry as he was home the next day anyway.

As the sun came up and everybody started to go about their day I realised how real this was and that I now needed to deal with things. I saw the doctor. She confirmed my miscarriage, made an appointment with a physiologist and lied to my boss, telling him I had the flu.

The weeks went on and I slowly came out of that dark place. My period returned and we had the green light to try again - this had me excited.

After just one month, I was pregnant again. Again, even before the test I knew it! I took the test and after seeing the positive sign I ran in to show my husband. Then, I instantly burst into tears. I was worried but excited. I was determined to be positive and make this time different.

I saw my OB as early as possible and scheduled in a 8 week scan. I was determined to do it all differently.

The weeks went past and I was feeling good. We had shared our news with a few friends and family.

I was 7 weeks and had had a couple of massive days at work and started to feel some light cramping. I put it down to doing too much but non the less, I went straight in for a scan.

This time, a heartbeat! I felt relieved. The technician said I was dating 6 weeks. I questioned her as I was confident on my dates. Heck, I knew exactly the time I was ovulating and conceived! She said not to worry as there was a heartbeat and all looked okay. I tried to put the dating issue behind me and not think about it. Again, I thought if I remained positive, everything had to be okay.

Then one day I came home from work and my husband and family were waiting outside of our house and something was off. We had an internal flood in our home and everything was ruined.

The house was unliveable for months and most of our possessions were ruined. It was devastating. Thank goodness for insurance.

Somehow I kept a positive attitude and kept saying to myself 'We may have lost our house but we are pregnant.' We moved in with my parents while the cleanup started on our house. This was such a stressful time. But I couldn't help thinking I was still lucky because I was pregnant.

Our 8 week scan came around and we felt excited. I lay on the table and the technician started looking at our baby. She said the dates didn't look right, the heartbeat was weak and she was sorry, I was going to miscarry.

This news hit me so hard. I felt like it winded me. I quickly got dressed and ran out to the car. I left my husband behind to deal with the paperwork. I didn't even think about how he was feeling. I rang Mum and again I couldn't talk. I couldn't even breathe. I then rang my OB and he saw us straight away. He confirmed my missed miscarriage and gave me a few options.

I decided to take the wait and see approach and let my body do it naturally. My OB was awesome and I am still grateful for his caring, compassionate bedside manner.

We went home to my parents and we just sat for hours in shock. Was this really happening again? We just lost our house! What the fuck was happening in this world for us to have to go through this again?

The next day I shared the news with our friends and family. From here I quickly went to a deep and dark place. I honestly thought I would feel this sad and somber for the rest of my life. This time I'd even let my self plan for our little girl's due date. I bought a couple of maternity items and truly started to plan ahead. Now it was all over and I was losing another baby.

The time passed and I slipped into a really bad headspace. I started to think I would never be able to carry a baby or be a Mum. All while I was still waiting to miscarry. The daily cramping was torturous. I was constantly worried I would start bleeding while I was at work or out.

I decided to share the news with my boss. He was surprisingly understandable as his wife had experienced miscarriages too. I kept it from my coworkers and quickly became a recluse. I was no longer my bright and happy self. I was a damaged shell and I was so broken inside.

Yet I still waited to miscarry. Everyday as I walked kilometres for exercise, I debated in my head as to have a D&C or wait it out. I tried acupuncture and herbs to try and bring on the miscarriage.

Finally one Friday afternoon at work the cramps got intense and I knew it was coming. I rang my OB and he prescribed some strong pain relief. I tried so hard to be brave and make it to the end of the day at work but I could hardly talk or walk from the pain.

That night back at my parents, where we were still living, I started to bleed. All over again I felt the emotions of a miscarriage. Of course, all this was happening while Ben was out at work. What was wrong with this world? I couldn't help but think I had done something terrible in a past life to have such awful things like this happen to me?

The cramping and pain was intense. Over the next 24hrs it worsened and I honestly felt like I was going to die - from both the physical and emotional pain. As things worsened I ended up in hospital and on a drip for pain relief. I couldn't believe I had to go through this all without my husband. We were both heartbroken.

To make matters worse I was put in the maternity unit as this is where I would receive the right care. I felt out of place. I felt like a burden. But most of all I felt lonely and gutted. I was in a place surrounded by women having babies. And here I was losing my second baby. Mum went home that evening and I was alone in the hospital room. Feeling like a failure. Alone and scared. And that evening, alone in my room, I went to the toilet and that's where I delivered my baby.

I was shocked. I panicked. I don't think I wanted to see her. It was too raw and real. All I wanted was my husband to hold me and he was so far away.

After my second miscarriage the recovery felt long and lonely. I saw a psychologist - on my own and with my husband. This process helped me to accept what happened. It also taught me that I didn't have to move on or get over these events, but learn to live with them as a part of my story. Later I would learn that there was no destiny or plan or God. That simply shit things happen to good people for no reason at all. Grief does not discriminate.

We finally moved back into our home and months passed and I obsessed over my cycle. Timing didn't work with my husbands time at home and I felt like I had taken two steps back. We booked a tropical holiday and I let my self relax and enjoy this holiday. My husbands shift changed and he was suddenly home at the right times. And then one month later, I was pregnant.

This time everything felt so clinical. I tried so hard to not get too excited, obsess or get attached. I rode a rollercoaster of emotions for the first trimester. I tried to give myself little milestones to make it through.

The first ultrasound was at 8 weeks and I felt so nervous. My OB performed the ultrasound and he was very quick to reassure me that our baby was dating spot on and with a strong heartbeat. I felt relief yet couldn't let go of the anxiety. I look back and don't know how I mentally made it to the 12 week mark, but I did.

On 14 November 2014 our first beautiful daughter was born. On 3 November 2016, her little sister joined her.

Megan Carlson

There are a number of reasons why I wanted to share Megan's story. She shares an experience that I've heard shared in the stories of countless other women. That is; not feeling like she was treated by doctors and nurses with enough empathy and understanding. Or being made to feel that losing a baby is 'not a big deal' because you were only x number of weeks.

Your loss, your baby is important. The way you feel about your baby is important. If you were made to feel any other way or treated as if your feelings were insignificant - that is not okay. Please read to the end of Megan's story, her final statement is profound and true.

Where do I even begin?

It was December 18, 2015 that we found out we were pregnant for the first time. My husband and I were over the moon; having kids is what we always dreamed of. From the minute the test turned positive, we starting planning and talking about the baby, and thinking of creative ways that we would tell our family. We were thrilled. Little did we know that the excitement and glow would quickly fade.

We knew that it was very early, but wanted to at least tell our immediate family. We took my parents out to breakfast and told them the exciting news, saying that our niece better watch out because there was another grandchild on the way. My parents were very happy.

For my in laws, my husband and I wanted to get creative. After our Christmas Eve party, we rushed to beat them home so we could set up our surprise. We ended up opening gifts that night due to my father in law having to work the next day. We saved our surprise for last. We told my in laws that their last present was somewhere in the kitchen. After minutes of searching, we decided to give them clues so they could find it.

My mother-in-law eventually opened the oven door and exclaimed, *'Who put a piece of bread in here?'* We all laughed and my father-in-law just looked at us and started crying.

He said, '*Are you serious?*'. Of course, he was the first one to get it.

My mother-in-law eventually put the pieces together and was overjoyed. My father-in-law kept saying, '*Oh my gosh, I can't believe it..*' Christmas was extra special that year.

On December 30, my husband and I left for 2 weeks for our Disney honeymoon. We had gotten married in August of that same year. We were so excited as we both had not been to Disney in over 20 years and we couldn't wait to relax and take everything in. Everything was perfect. The Florida weather was beautiful. We were so excited to be expecting.

On the second day we were there I started to notice some discharge. I had no idea what it was at the time, but I was freaking out. I told my husband and, being who he is, he just remained calm and tried to calm me down. I was in tears. I was so close to telling him that I wanted to go to the hospital just to make sure that everything was okay.

We returned to our hotel room and tried to relax. I kept telling myself that we had had a very long day the day before and did a lot of walking and it was probably just the usual spotting. By this time, I was going on 2 months.

The spotting continued on and off for 3 or 4 days. Each time it stopped I was relieved. But then it would come back and I was back to freaking out. We spent 5 nights on Disney property and then it was time for 4 nights on the Disney Cruise. I was feeling better by the time we got on the boat and tried to enjoy myself. This was my honeymoon after all and we hadn't had a vacation in years, I tried to take everything in and get my mind off the spotting.

I was feeling better until I went to the bathroom. After I wiped, I noticed brown, stringy mucus discharge. My freaking out went from nonexistent to through the roof. I immediately called my OB/GYN at the time and talked to her medical assistant. She gave me the news that I feared the most, '*I think you are having a miscarriage.*'

My heart sank and I tried to hold back the tears as best I could. She told me that I needed to seek medical attention right away. Well, it's not that easy when you are on a cruise ship that's about to set sail to the Bahamas! I tried to remain calm. I called my husband in from our verandah and burst into tears. I told him everything that the MA had told me. He held me as I cried and we tried to figure things out. Thankfully there was a doctor on the ship who was available. We went to see her and all she could do was a pelvic exam and tell me that my uterus was closed.

She suggested that I go to a medical centre when we docked in Nassau the next day. She was able to make the appointment for us and told us that our transportation would be taken care of. As much as I wanted time to slow down and to enjoy my honeymoon with my husband, I was anxious to see that doctor in Nassau. The time couldn't come fast enough and when it finally did, I wished for all that time back. We were taken to a women's medical centre and, to be honest, I was scared, not only for my baby, but for my husband and I. I was thankful that we didn't have to walk through the streets and that we were taken straight to the centre.

I had to fill out some paperwork as usual and then we began to wait. They called me in and I had to give them a urine sample. After that, the nurse took us to the room where we waited some more. Finally the doctor came in and as I had feared; the doctor was a man. I don't know why, but I've never been comfortable around male gynaecologists. I've always seen a woman doctor. But I had no choice in that moment.

I just wanted him to hurry up with the ultrasound so I could see what was going on. The ultrasound had to be transvaginal due to me being so early on in the pregnancy. According to the app on my phone, I was supposed to be 7 weeks and 5 days. The doctor measured the baby at 5 weeks 5 days. 2 weeks behind. My heart dropped. My husband thought that maybe I had ovulated later and that I wasn't as far along as I thought I was.

The doctor was able to find a heartbeat on the tiny little bean that we saw on the screen. I'll never forget that beautiful sound; it was music to my ears at 150(?) beats per minute. The doctor told us that the heart could have just started beating or that the baby was dying.

I don't even want to get into how rude and unsympathetic this doctor was. He had the worst bedside manner and could not have been more unsympathetic towards us. He basically told me that I had a threatened miscarriage and there was nothing I could do. He said *'If it happened, it happened.'*

We were able to get a picture of our little bean before we left. In Nassau, they did not accept my health insurance because we are from the United Stated. We had to pay $740 out of pocket. Nothing like adding to the misery and pain of our whole experience. The whole time I kept thinking to myself, *"We should have just gone to an ER before we boarded the ship. Ugh"*.
We finished out our honeymoon as best we could and I tried to enjoy every minute even though it was hard and I was constantly worried. I can't remember when the discharge stopped, but it was before we got home.

I was feeling a little bit better about the situation, but not much. My OB/GYN wouldn't see me until I was at least 8 weeks. My initial appointment with them was the Friday after we got home and the day before my birthday.

It wasn't very much of an appointment and I was not too happy about that. All they did was have me pee in a cup, go over my entire health history, take some blood, and gave me a folder with a ton of information about pregnancy and what to expect along the way.

I was told that I needed to have more blood draw on Sunday to check my HCG levels. I did not see my doctor at all, nor did I have an ultrasound. I left upset and not happy with how I was treated. I tried to enjoy my birthday weekend with my friends.

On Sunday I had my blood drawn and then began the waiting. I was told that my doctor's office would call the next day and let me know the results. I called in sick to work on Monday and didn't receive a call from my doctor's office. I tried calling them and left a message, but I didn't get a response. More worry and waiting. They finally called me late Tuesday afternoon and explained that my levels had dropped, but not by much.

They wanted me to come in as soon as they had an opening which was in 2 WEEKS! I was thinking, '*What the hell? Why can't you get me in now?*' I couldn't wait two more weeks! I was very frustrated and upset to say the least.

The next day the office called me again. They said they had an opening at noon if I was able to make it. I told them I would be there no matter what. I explained to my boss what was happening. She also wasn't as sympathetic as I thought she would be. I did what I had to do in order to leave on time. At the time I had over an hour drive to and from work and the whole time I was praying that I made it safely to the doctors. The car couldn't go fast enough and the miles seemed twice as long as they normally did, but I made it. I got there and waited some more. My husband showed up right as they called me in. It was finally time to find out what was going on. It seemed to take forever before the doctor finally came in. This was my first time meeting her and she appeared very nice and cheerful. She was very positive as soon as she walked in and explained what I could expect over the next nine months. I just nodded as she talked; feeling that I already knew the baby was gone. She needed to use the transvaginal wand due to the pregnancy being so early. I couldn't see the screen but I knew as soon as I saw her face that it was officially over. I had miscarried and my body wasn't naturally flushing out the remains. She eventually showed me what she found; a little empty sac with nothing in it. Our baby was gone.

The doctor explained that the pregnancy had probably ended weeks ago and my body had absorbed our tiny bean of a baby, but the sac remained. She went on to explain the mystery of miscarriage, the hows and the whys, and all the stuff that I didn't feel like hearing at that moment.

She also explained different options I could take. We could wait 2-3 cycles and start trying again or I could go back on the pill for a while and go from there. There was also a third option, but I don't remember what it was.

I had decided to go back on the pill for at least 3 months and be off it for 3 months and then we would start trying again in June/July. At the time, she prescribed misoprostol aka the 'abortion pill' to help my body clean out my uterus. I had to take that for 5 nights in a row and I cried every time I had to take it. It didn't help that I also had to finish out the work week; being at work was the last place I wanted to be. I felt like I couldn't do my job because I was distracted, distant, uninterested.

I felt useless, like I failed. I felt like I could've done something to prevent this when in reality there was nothing I could do or that could've been done. I waited for the pain, the cramps, the blood, but it never came. I had light spotting for one day and that was it until 3 weeks later when I experienced the most unimaginable pain I had ever experienced. This lasted for about 2-3 weeks and each time I went to the bathroom and saw blood, my heart broke all over again.

Each time was a reminder of my baby that I'd lost. I was devastated. It didn't help that I had to attend a baby shower a few weeks after that. It took everything in me to hold back the tears. I bawled my eyes out to my husband when I got home and he held me and told me that everything was going to be okay.

After everything was said and done, we told our parents and siblings, everyone whom we initially told. They all felt bad, of course, but what do you say in a situation like this? I wouldn't even know what to say myself!

Afterwards I seemed to notice baby related things everywhere and each time I would cry. The baby showers and pregnancy announcements didn't help either and my longing for my lost baby grew and grew.

I decided to seek out counselling because I was feeling very depressed and not like myself. I needed help to cope and talk to someone who could help me through my sadness. I can't say enough good things about my counsellor. I loved our sessions and each time I went I felt so much better afterward. Talking with her really helped me to heal and deal with my situation and realise that I wasn't alone (even though I felt like I was).

She was very warm and comforting and helped me overcome the hurdles of feelings that miscarriage brings with it. It was a long time before my husband and I had sex again and the first time we did, I cried. It really helped talking about this to my counsellor and we eventually got back to our normal routine and my libido returned.

During this time, I let the world know what had happened because I was tired of pretending to be happy and putting on a show in front of those who didn't know. I was tired of the act and I wasn't ashamed of what had happened. Telling the world helped my healing process because I didn't have to explain why I was feeling down or looking sad or didn't show up to family gatherings. Everyone knew and understood. They were all very supportive.

I felt like I was getting better with each day that passed and was trying to become more positive about a future pregnancy. One miscarriage was enough heartache for me for a lifetime. It was mid-late April when I was on my final pack of birth control. I finished out my off week and was so happy to be done with the pill. I had downloaded some apps on my phone in order to track my ovulation to be sure that we avoided sex during those times.

On the second weekend in May I was attending my cousin's bridal shower with my Mom and 1 year old niece. My niece was sick in the car and we didn't bring extra clothes so I had to run to Target and get her a new outfit. The whole day felt rushed and I was flushed by the time I got home. My breast started feeling tender and I thought that maybe my period was due and from the looks of my calendar it should be coming very soon.

On a whim and womanly instinct, I took a pregnancy test. I didn't even need to wait the full three minutes; the test turned positive right away. I started to hyperventilate and pace the bathroom floor. I was in shock. I kept telling myself, *'No, it's too early. I'm not ready. It's not time. This can't be true.'*

We had hardly had sex and I'd literally just stopped the pill so I didn't think that I could get pregnant so easily and so fast. I came down the stairs crying with the positive test in my hand. I showed my husband and he was more excited than I was. I was in tears and he was all smiles. I told him that I wasn't ready and it wasn't time and that I couldn't go through losing another baby.

After I stopped crying, I called my doctor to make yet another appointment. I knew what to expect this time around with having to go through that stupid initial appointment again with the history and folder and blah, blah, blah. We decided not to tell anyone this time in fear of going through another miscarriage again. I told my boss though, in case, god forbid I should suffer another miscarriage.

I tried to remain positive and to be happy about this pregnancy, but it was hard for me. I was worried from the minute the test turned positive. I prayed every night. I tried to take even better care of myself. I avoided anything and everything that could even possibly harm the baby.

Every time I went to the bathroom I was terrified that I would see the spotting again, but it never came. April turned to May and May turned to June and with each passing day I was getting more positive that this pregnancy was going to work out. We were going to get our baby this time around. I counted down the days until my first ultrasound which wasn't scheduled until I was almost 10 weeks, another fact I was upset about. I called almost every other day to see if there was an opening or cancellation so I could get in earlier. It was at this time that I got the feeling that my doctor's office didn't really care about me.

I started to realise that my symptoms weren't as strong as they had been a week or two before and this scared me. I didn't have morning sickness this time around, but my breasts stopped hurting, my heartburn went away, and I barely had any symptoms at all anymore. I explained my worry and lack of symptoms to the nurse and she told me to just relax, that symptoms come and go and everyone was different. Even so, they couldn't get me in any earlier. I had just wait.

It was June 14 and I was at work when I realised that I felt aching, period-like cramps. I thought that maybe I hadn't had enough water the day before so I made sure that I drank water like crazy. The cramps continued for most of the day and I thought that maybe I was walking too much. When I got home I went to the bathroom and there it was.

That brown, mucous discharge had returned. My heart dropped. I ran downstairs and told my husband. I told him that I wanted to go to the emergency room right away. He was reluctant to take me, but I told him that couldn't relax until I knew what was going on. We got to the ER and they took me in right away. They needed a urine sample, of course, and wanted to make sure that I wasn't bleeding otherwise they would need to put a catheter in. They gave me three wipes to wipe myself three separate times. On the third time I wiped, there was every expectant mother's worst fear; bright red blood with some stringy discharge. I knew right then and there that it was over. I was so shocked I didn't know what to do. They had to put the catheter in me to get the urine sample. They did a pelvic exam and ultrasound. The pelvic exam showed I had some brown blood/discharge, but not too much. The ultrasound measured the baby at about 5 weeks 4 days; *way behind*. I should have been at least 8 weeks. No heart beat was detected, but the doctor said that wasn't unusual because the pregnancy was very early.

My HCG levels also weren't as high as they should have been for 8 weeks. The ER doctor was very positive and said that everything lined up with me being 5 weeks 4 days. He was so different from the doctor in the Bahamas. I appreciated his kindness and positivity. They sent us home and I text my boss saying that I needed at least one day to rest and then I could return to work. That night was uneventful. I didn't see any blood or discharge. The next day the cramps started again and I knew these feelings all too well. I only felt comfortable sitting on the toilet and in the bath tub.

The process had started. I was losing the baby and my body was ready to get rid of everything. My period was due that day and I realised that I was probably having a missed miscarriage.

Everything passed that night and all the feelings and depression came back full force. I called my doctor the next day and they were miraculously able to get me in to talk to my doctor. Thankfully I was scheduled to see my counsellor that next day as well.

My doctor's appointment was uneventful. They drew blood before I went in and confirmed that I'd miscarried. My levels had dropped rapidly from the ER visit until now. Nothing new was said that we hadn't heard the first time around. She prescribed me some pills for pain and sent me on my way. Nothing more, nothing less.

I brought my husband to my counselling session and my counsellor knew immediately what had happened. It was the best idea to bring my husband. We were able to talk about feelings and the loss and everything in between. She was so helpful and I was glad that I was able to talk about this miscarriage right away. I couldn't believe that this had happened for the second time. I felt like I failed yet again, like my body was betraying me because I couldn't carry a baby. I couldn't do my job as a woman because I kept losing babies. It was as if the whole process was repeating itself. That Sunday was Father's Day and I decided to acknowledge my husband and tell the world that we now had two babies in heaven.

Nothing will ever be the same. My due dates came and went and it has already been a year since we lost our first baby. We lost two babies within 5 months in 2016 and I feel like that's enough heartache to last a lifetime. Ever since our second loss, we haven't been pregnant. We haven't been tracking anything, but it doesn't seem as easy as it did before. There have been more baby showers, pregnancies and birth announcements and they all hit me hard.

I know the triggers will always be there, but damn it's so hard some days to feel happy for these people and not feel sorry for myself. We went shopping for a baby shower in August, right around the time I was supposed to be due with our first baby and I broke down and cried in the middle of the baby aisle at Target. I couldn't do it. It wasn't fair. It's not fair.

I want children more than anything in my life and it seems that I'm not able to have them. I want to damn all these people who make getting pregnant look so easy. Why is it so hard for me? Will this happen a third time? How could I go through everything again?

As of now, we have started trying again. It's so hard for me to pinpoint my ovulation and I'm already getting frustrated with the whole process. Some days I want to throw my hands up in air and say '*Fuck it all, I don't care, if it happens, it happens.*' But it's so hard for me to not track anything. I feel like it's an obsession.

Most of my friends and family members are having their second and third babies and here I am with no living children. Hoping, praying, crying, and trying desperately to have our first. All I can do is put in God's hand and try to believe that it will happen when the time is right. I just hope that is sooner rather than later.

You never forget your babies. What could have been. Who they would look like. What their personality might be. I'll always wonder who my children would have been. I just hope that we will eventually get our rainbow baby and many more babies after that. I found this prayer that I really love.

Dear Lord, I would have loved to hold my baby in my arms and tell them about you, but since I didn't get the chance, will you hold them in your arms and tell them about me?

Have faith, my fellow mothers. Everything will be alright. Know that you are not alone. Everything is always okay in the end. **If it's not okay, then it's not the end.**

Alison

I have to admit I struggled to read Alison's story when she first sent it to me. The way she describes her experiences so honestly felt confronting. Often when we read about loss the graphic parts are glossed over or avoided completely. Our own experience of miscarriage or stillbirth can feel traumatic in comparison. I leave Alison's story here unedited, because I think there is value in reading stories that so accurately reflect the graphic nature of our own.

In 2014 we were living with my parents whilst we were building our home. We had 2 children already and another on the way. I woke one night at 8 weeks pregnant to a bleed. It was thick and so red.

I cried and cried and rang the hospital. They said there is nothing they could do but if I wanted to come in, I could. My heart sank. There wasn't anything to do. A miscarriage at this stage meant nothing. Just a statistic. We went in, 2 beautiful daughter in tow. We sat patiently in the waiting room for ages.

Finally a doctor came out and did a scan - there was a heartbeat! And a big cloud beside it. He said it could have possibly been a twin.

Another scan was booked for the following Monday and again the heartbeat was strong.

Everything went well until 4 weeks later when I had another bleed. This time there was cramping. *My heart sank.* I didn't have cramping before. I knew this was it. I felt sick and so tired. I went to sleep and when I woke I had massive pains. I felt like I had to go to the toilet.As I sat on the toilet I had a massive urge to push.

As I pushed I could see our baby coming out. It was stuck and no matter how hard I pushed it was still connected to something inside me. I felt like I was going to faint so I had to break the umbilical cord with my fingers. I collapsed to the ground crying.

My baby was in the toilet drowning. My Mum rushed over and went to get my Dad to take me to the hospital (Scott, my husband, was at work). I couldn't leave my baby in the toilet alone, cold and drowning. I fished him out and put him in an ice cream container.

At 12.5 weeks our baby was so long. He had that white clear looking skin. And fingers and toes. His eyes were indented and he had a little mouth. It broke my heart.

The next few months we discovered a 6 x 6 cyst. We also had 13 weekly HCG tests, waiting for my levels to come down. Finally another doctor saw the cyst, tested my ca125 levels and then did a Roma screening.

They thought I had cancer, so the cyst had to come out.

My miscarriage was in August and finally in February the cyst and one fallopian tube was removed. It was non-cancerous.

I blamed myself. It was winter and when we had the first bleed I was waking in hot sweats because I was overheating from the blankets and all the clothes I had on. Looking back I never felt 100% right throughout that pregnancy. I wasn't sick enough.

We started to try again. It took forever and with one less fallopian tube I worried we would never fall pregnant. By December we started talking IVF or AI.

On Christmas morning I took a pregnancy test. I didn't look at the stick properly at first and thought it was a no. When I looked later - I realised it was positive!

On boxing day we did the second test. A definite positive. We were so excited and quickly booked in our 6 week scan to make sure bub wasn't in my remaining tube and we got to see a little heartbeat. I was sent home to continue on my way. Every now and then my morning sickness would go away. I was worried this one wasn't right either.

At 9.5 weeks I started to bleed, than came the cramps. I knew it was over. I bawled when bub come out. It was nowhere near as physically painful but it was so hard. I got the baby out, it just was so floppy.

Mentally I was hurting. My heart was now stuck with the 2 babies I have here and the 2 babies that were gone. Our first went just after my Grandma died, so I knew she was up there looking after our baby. Our 2nd came after my Grumpy, Uncle and Scott's Pop had passed so I knew that baby was being well looked after too. We'd experienced so much death in 2 years. I found myself asking - *'Why me? Why 2? Am I that bad of a Mum?'*

I started to blame myself again. At the kid's gymnastics class that week I had gotten really hot. Maybe that caused it? I grieved and cried.

I didn't know what to do. Babies due around the same time as our first miscarriage were 1 now. I know it's not a race, but bloody hell. Here we were with 2 miscarriages.

My husband vowed to be there this time. Grief is so hard though. We both lost our babies. Yet we deal with it so differently I would cry and be sad for months after and then all of a sudden he would break down.

I googled everything trying to find out why it had happened. A friend introduced me to positive thinking. She told me I needed to learn to trust my body again.

So I did.

My hormones settled and I worked on trusting it would be okay. I told myself that *'My body can do this'*. I felt internally happy again. But god those hormones are hard.

At the end of September we found out we were expecting again. I was scared but kept repeating my mantra. *'I have this. My body has this. It knows what to do.'*

I was nauseous most of the day. My breasts swelled 2 sizes. My belly was bloating up quickly *'My body has this'* I thought. At night I struggled to get comfortable feeling like I could vomit. This was what I normally experienced. We had a scan at 6 and 8 weeks and decided to do another one at 10 just in case. We went for our 10 week scan. I emptied my bladder and the doctor lined up for our first external scan.

He put the thing on my belly on the 13th of December. Christmas was less than 2 weeks away. I had stopped feeling as sick the last few days, but was still a bit nauseous. There was no heartbeat. He looked and looked. Our baby measured 9w 3d. I knew this was bad.

I felt like screaming *'Just do the internal! Get a closer look!'*

Finally he said. *'I am just having trouble finding the heartbeat I will do an internal.'*

With this he left the room to call in the attendant to supervise. I held my husband's hand and cried. I told him our baby is dead. He hadn't seen the 9w 3d measurement so just thought we were looking for a heartbeat.

'How could I not have noticed our baby died?' I thought to myself. The doctor came back in. He looked and looked. No heartbeat.

I wanted to scream at him *'You will not find a heartbeat! It is dead.'*

Finally he said, *'I am very sorry but your baby has died.'*

Those words are so final. I had worked so hard at keeping cool. Wetting myself with water on hot days whilst people thought I was crazy. The girls were at a friends place. Straight away we booked in for a curette. I wanted this thing out.

Next morning I was to have the operation. I cried and cried. *'Why us!?'* I had this dead thing inside me and I felt like tomorrow could not come quick enough.

I cried as I waited but smiled at the nurses that would come and check on me. We got a photo of our baby. I felt horrible I never got to tell him I loved him. Because this was our third loss he was sent for chromosome testing. He was a boy (we have 2 girls and as much as we are happy, it would have been a bit cool to have a boy too). There were no chromosomal problems found.
I felt like it was my body's fault. *'I am lacking something.'* I thought. *'There was nothing wrong with our baby. I killed our baby.'*

On the way home. I spoke out loud. I knew that if I didn't I would later blame myself again.

'This isn't my fault or my body's. If I had known I was lacking something I would have taken whatever it was to fix the situation, I would love a baby and would take anything for it.'

My doctor gave me Q10, extra folate and herbal drugs to take from day 3 to day 10 of my cycle. I felt like we were finally doing something this time.

He thought my uterine wall lining was too thin so when my babies attached they were too close to the vein. It bleeds and then stops bub being able to grow and continue to attach properly.

I had always hoped I would have all our babies by 30. But here I was at 31 and still trying.

We had various announcements over this time. A friend who'd had 2 bubs and 2 miscarriages all around same times, was due at the same time as we would have been and another friend was due with twins.

Everyone has their own life but those announcements felt like a jagged knife in my heart. I often blame myself, our business, our house, the fancy things in our life. If I knew it would help, I would given it all up for our chance to have another baby.

Our marriage suffered after our third loss. We didn't talk as much and both just wanted to zone out. I hoped deep down he didn't blame me. This was the hardest few years of my life. The grief was so raw at this time. When you have another miscarriage you grieve again for your other children, all in heaven together.

I started seeing a Naturopath and Iridologist. He said my miscarriages had to do with my pituitary gland being out of balance. He gave me hundreds of dollars of medication to be taken over the next few months.

I started with the liver detox. 2 months of migraines followed. It was intense. Then medication to restore my liver and fix my pituitary gland.

Finally we were able to try again. I also went to see a Kinesiologist to clear my mind of negative thoughts. We worked on cleaning my mind and focusing on telling my body I could carry another baby full term.

I was so, so scared. But I needed to try and my heart ached for another baby. Scott was really keen to try one more time.

One Tuesday before Fathers Day I was feeling ill so peed on a stick. My period was not due 'til the following Monday. I couldn't believe it! A beautiful faint line came up!

I rang and made an appointment and showed the stick to Scott on Father's Day. This time all the grandparents found out Father's Day too. We decided that we'd tell them all later anyway, so may as well enjoy whatever time we have.

Glorious morning sickness ensued. I was doing progesterone pessaries morning and night and feeling nauseous all day long. It was dreadful but so comforting. Morning sickness means a healthy baby! I couldn't stand the smell of Scott! I nearly kicked him out of bed so many times.

We planned to have fortnightly scans from 6 weeks. At 9 weeks, I started to feel less nauseous. All the normal things wouldn't kick it back in. I rang my Obstetrician crying. He told me to come in for a scan.

I went there convinced there would be no heartbeat. But we heard a beautifully strong heartbeat.

We went home relieved. At 12 weeks we had a test that looks for any chromosome issues. My body has issues absorbing folate, though this apparently wasn't the issue with my miscarriages. We finally got to tell our beautiful girls. They were so excited and smiled ear to ear.

I never stopped worrying throughout our entire pregnancy. I would listen to positive mantras. I rested way more than I ever had before. Our baby was growing amazingly well and was getting bigger and bigger.

Our beautiful baby girl was welcomed into the world on May 8. I cried as I held our gorgeous girl. I felt so thankful and still somewhat surprised I got the chance to meet her.

Adjusting to babyhood after 6 years has been hard. I've had a lot of mastitis and questions from others about if she was an accident. I'd definitely gotten used to getting to places quicker and just being able to do more. But I wouldn't swap her for the world.

Sheryl Young

The way I connected with Sheryl feels like it was meant to be. During the process of self-publishing this book I realised I needed to hire someone to complete the cover design. I searched Instagram using random hashtags for artists and came across Sheryl's work. I sent her a message and knew she was the right person when she replied straight away saying that she'd practiced some of my fertility yoga classes on Youtube.

I knew I wanted watercolour and black ink, but the rest of the info I gave her was pretty vague. We talked through the idea of the woman's face and of including flowers as a nod to the title, but that was about it. I also sent her a very early draft of the book to give her an idea of the message I was trying to convey. A few weeks later she sent me a rough sketch of the cover design. I'm not exaggerating when I tell you I could have used that as the cover right then and there.

As we continued to work together on the cover Sheryl opened up about her own journey and I encouraged her to share her story here. Not only because it felt right, but also because her story speaks to truths that the other stories in this collection haven't touched on. I believe that in the process of conceiving our babies we experience grief of many types. Getting your period yet again, or going through an IVF round is a loss. It's a loss of all the hopes and dreams you had for this baby that feels as real to you as one in your arms.

When Bettina shared an earlier draft of her book with me, I honestly had so many moments where I felt like I was reading my own thoughts. Even though my story is a little different to hers, I felt the same multitude of emotions with my experience of loss.

My husband and I have been 'trying' on and off for the last 8 years. We're both heading towards our late thirties now and I feel this overwhelming sense that time is running out. Unlike the other ladies who have shared their stories, I have never fallen pregnant. I have never had a positive result, natural or with IVF. I can only dream of the day where I take a pregnancy test and it comes up with two lines or the day that a nurse calls me and says *'Congratulations, you're going to be a mum!.'*

That would be amazing and surreal. After so many unsuccessful cycles, a part of me is making peace with the fact that we may never have a family. This is the loss that I'm grieving. I feel like there is a small hole in my heart now. It's not enough to completely stop it from beating but I know it's there. If it never gets filled, my husband and I will no doubt still live an enjoyable life, just the two of us.

I'll eventually learn to live with it and we'll be okay, family or no family. I say this to myself a lot these days. Some days it's easy to believe, other days it's more challenging.

It's funny to think that my husband was ready to start trying for a family early on in our relationship but I was like *'no way, you're crazy man'*. I was still studying at university and I didn't feel anywhere near ready. I naively thought we had all the time in the world back then. It didn't even occur to me that we would have troubles conceiving when I finally felt everything aligned for us to start a family.

We spent a lot of years trying naturally and seeing different naturopaths and holistic doctors to help us increase our chances.

Frustratingly, I wasn't falling pregnant and it was becoming apparent that we were going to need to go down the IVF route. In the midst of all that, I was diagnosed with latent tuberculosis and I had to go through a course of heavy antibiotics which meant another setback for us.

It felt like we were trying to swim upstream and it really made me question whether I was trying to force something that clearly wasn't meant to be.

Meanwhile, all of my friends were falling pregnant left, right and centre. I felt like such a failure. Every time I received someone else's good news - I wanted to be happy but it triggered so many negative thoughts and emotions because it felt so unfair.

Why not me?
Was there something wrong with me?
Was I a bad person?
Was I not worthy?
Was I not fit to be a parent?

Was my relationship with my husband not good enough?

To top it off, everyone had advice or a story of a sister, a family member, a friend, a work colleague who tried this, who did that and they fell pregnant straight away. I do recognise that people had good intentions and wanted to comfort me but it did the opposite. It just made me feel worse about myself.

Relaxing holidays, changing my diet, holistic healers, more exercise, less exercise, hypnotherapy, fertility crystals, you name it I tried it. I even had a family member pass away a week or two after my embryo transfer (not that I planned or caused this). I mention it because as soon as it happened, someone said to me *'Oh, you know what they say, someone has to pass away for a new soul to be born, it's going to happen for you soon!'*.

It's disheartening when it's never you.

I went into the first fertility treatment with such high hopes but every negative cycle chipped away at that. I felt at breaking point last year when I had back to back embryo transfers, all with negative results.

It was heartbreaking.

When I talk to people about IVF, they instantly bring up financial costs. While that can be a pain point, I mean seriously, we could have gone on a few awesome holidays with the amount we've spent (not to mention the sessions of reiki healing, herbal medication and acupuncture that I was going to on a regular basis to support the process). It was more the emotional, physical and emotional toll that bothered me.

I was becoming severely depressed and I couldn't find the joy in anything anymore. My life became all about IVF and falling pregnant.

I didn't really see friends or go out all that much last year, in part because of all the random clinic appointments and because I felt too tired and sad. I was a shadow of myself. Every conversation I had felt hollow and I had to fight back tears. I felt like I was constantly disappointing family and friends.

As well as that, I wasn't really coping with work, I felt extremely drained every day and I couldn't focus, which of course made me feel like even more of a failure at life.

At the moment, we're still on our IVF journey albeit on a much needed break. I've given myself permission to heal. My priority is to cultivate a more positive mindset.

We have one last frozen embryo to transfer before my husband and I close this chapter of our lives. A huge part of me has been wounded too many times to think that I'll meet my baby with this final attempt.

I was going to have the transfer done earlier in the year with the attitude of *'Let's just get this thing over and done with so we can move on with our lives.'*

However, I caught myself and thought what is the point if I go into the procedure with already a dismissive 'whatever' mentality. I wholeheartedly want to approach this last transfer with faith in myself, in the universe and in the process.

I want to give it a fighting chance. I think time is the biggest healer, so I'm going to take as much of it as I need to replenish my spirit and energy. When the time comes, I want to lean into feelings of love and have an open heart, even if it means it might get hurt again.

'You've got to trust yourself. Be gentle with yourself. And listen to yourself. You're the only person who can get you through this now. You're the only one who can survive your story, the only one who can write your future. All you've got to do, when you're ready, is stand up, (and begin again.)' - Tessa Shaffer

PART THREE - ADVICE FROM A FRIEND

"...until the body, or the heart, or the bank was broken, they didn't know who they were, what they felt, or what they wanted. Before their descent into the darkness, they took more than they gave, or they were numb, or full of fear or blame or self-pity. In their most broken moments they were brought to their knees; they were humbled; they were opened. And later, as they pulled the pieces back together, they discovered a clearer sense of purpose and a new passion for life." - Elisabeth Lesser

This section includes the advice I would like to have known in the early days and weeks after my losses. I have hesitated over whether to share these words here with you.

Each loss is so individual and personal and I know that something that would have helped me, may make you feel angry or hurt at the mere thought of it.

If you have a strong negative reaction to anything written in this section I would like to encourage you to take some time to sit with those emotions and decide for yourself how *you* feel them.

My words and ideas are most definitely not gospel. It is my intention that you receive the advice that I share here as if it were from a friend. It was written with love, but please *take it or leave it.*

EARLY DAYS AFTER LOSS

Let everything unnecessary fall away.

The first few days, weeks and months after each loss are the absolute worst. You're still physically recovering. Your heart is broken. All the plans you had for the next few months and years, through the pregnancy and with your baby are gone. Instead you're left with this great big void of nothingness, and no way to fill it.

In those first few months after losing each baby I felt like I was underwater. I could see all of the other people and hear what they were saying but it was like life was muffled for meaning. I couldn't connect with anyone or anything in the same way that I used to.

I no longer cared about plans we had to renovate the bathroom. Things that had felt like a big deal before, things that were important to me before, no longer mattered. I found myself feeling like '*Who cares about any of this when my baby is dead?*'.

I used to worry about the size of my bum and it being bigger than I thought it should be, but afterwards - '*Who cares about any of that when my baby is dead?*'

I used to worry about the house being a mess, or not having enough money to buy the new car we thought we needed or that my hair had started going grey.

But now? '*Who cares about any of THAT when my baby is dead?*'

After our losses life felt trivial and meaningless. I started questioning why any of it had mattered to me in the first place. It was like I'd woken up to a new way of seeing the world. One where everything was held up to the fact that my baby was dead and in contrast to THAT, nothing mattered.

At first this new perspective felt overwhelming. You can easily venture down into 'why bother?' territory and that is a scary place to be.

If that's you at the moment allow yourself to move slowly through these feelings. If you feel like doing nothing but bingeing on Netflix, then do exactly that. If you need to spend a few weeks moping in bed, or around the house, then do that. If you want to throw yourself straight back into normal life, do that.

If you feel the desire to jump into something new as a distraction, then do that (Although can I suggest probably hold off on making any life-altering decisions at this point. New creative project or hobbies = good. Throwing away an entire career = maybe wait until you're out of the fresh grief stage for big decisions like that).

Ultimately though there are no rules to how you 'should' operate in the early days after you've lost a baby.

Personally I found that I needed to hermit myself for a little bit longer after each consecutive loss before I was ready to return to the world. It was like each loss knocked me a little bit harder, and I needed more time to put the pieces back together before I could return to regular life.

After each loss I found that I let more and more of my life fall away. I stopped caring so much about what everyone thought. I let go of work that I didn't really love. I let go of friends who felt like hard work. I became really particular about how I spent my time.

It became really clear what was truly important to me. My husband. My boys. My family. My close friends. My writing. My work in this space. *Me.*

Take your time after each loss to let what needs to fall away, and graciously do exactly that. Don't bother trying to hold onto friendships that are struggling under the weight of grief. Grieving is emotionally and energetically draining, keep the little energy you do have for looking after yourself and those people in your life who are important to you.

Most people won't know what to say. Many will definitely say the wrong awkward thing. Others will be downright offensive. Know that this is often not their intention and most people think they are being helpful. No one can understand your grief if they haven't been there themselves. Forgive them for that.

At the same time, you can allow this process to help you cull those from your life that no longer belong in it. Those who are no longer prepared to stand beside you in your darkest times.

This experience asks those closest to us to step up, and you will quickly learn who is up to the task. Don't waste your energy trying to hold onto those who are not there for you. If there ever was a time to be selfish and look after yourself first, this is it.

You don't necessarily need to make rash decisions about getting rid of people or things from your life though. To be honest, even some of the most important people in your life are going to say dumb things to you when you're grieving for a baby.

Some of the things they say will sting badly and possibly make you question why you ever liked them in the first place. This doesn't mean you have to get rid of every person who is a little challenged when it comes to finding the right things to say or do, (because this could be pretty much everyone). It does mean that you get a free pass to not waste your energy on anyone who you don't find helpful to your healing at the time.

Spend time with those friends and family members who fill you back up when you're running low and those who don't deplete your energy when you see them. Eventually, you'll find that those who you haven't put energy into will either fall away on their own, or if they're meant to, they will return to your life in a new helpful way.

You may also find that your work is no longer as meaningful to you after losing a baby. If you can financially afford to, perhaps this is the time to take a bit of a break so that you can focus on healing.

Or if you can't afford to take time off, maybe you can take a bit of a mental break from work. If you're usually the type to give 150% and to take home the worries of your day with you, allow yourself to do just the bare minimum. Give what you need to get the job done but save your energy for healing and focusing on those things that do feel important to you.

Look after your physical health

While it can be tempting to drown your sorrows in all the quick fixes, now is not the time to put your body under any more stress than it already is. Try to keep up with at least some good healthy habits at this time, despite how you probably feel. You will most likely not feel like doing this; but know that good nutrition, lots of water, comforting rituals to encourage sleep and regular movement will help your body to process the grief that is permeating in your heart, mind and womb.

If you have no motivation to cook, order in pre-prepared meals or ask for support from friends and family. (They'll probably also love having a practical way to help you, rather than just popping round with their awkward words and being unsure what to do.)

Sleep may feel impossible or you may want to stay in bed all day long, but you'll probably also feel more exhausted than you ever have in your life. You get a free pass to do whatever works in the days immediately after losing a baby. After a few weeks though, it will help to find a bit of a routine around your sleep again.

If falling asleep is the problem (because your mind takes over and has you thinking all the things) create a little bedtime ritual with a warm bath, tea and reading until your eyes are ready to fall out of your head. Try to read an actual book. (Reading on your phone is less likely to help you fall asleep soundly.) Don't read anything on babies or loss. Pick up something trashy, easy to read.

Exercise is probably the last thing you feel like doing and of course, until you're physically well enough - continue to sloth away. Once you're able to though, movement is a great way to help the body move feelings of grief.

Our bodies store our emotions and experiences within them. Unless we give these experiences a way to express themselves we will carry them in our body for many years, often without even being aware of it.

Walking and yoga are great places to start, although I also found that on my worst days running (even though I actually despise it) worked well to shift the really big negative emotions I was feeling.

Movement also gives you a nice big endorphin high which will help to lift your mood. It honestly doesn't really matter what you choose to do though. Try not to overthink it and just move in a way that feels good for you.

Even if it feels at first like you're just going through the motions of these healthy habits, do the best you can to help your body to heal.

On a practical level looking after your physical health is often the one thing you can do, amidst a whole lot of 'nothing helps.' While it of course won't fix your grieving heart, it will help you to eventually find the energy again to start healing the heartache. When you're ready.

Avoid Isolation

I don't know why, but we always assume that we are unique in our experiences. We feel like no one else feels the same way we do and that what we are going through is somehow different, greater or lesser than others. We believe that we are alone in our failures, our bad habits and our longings. Rather than admitting how we're feeling - we try to pretend that we're okay. We pretend that we've got it all together, and that we're not suffering.

This is how we behave about almost everything else, so it's not surprising that when it comes to miscarriage and stillbirth, we accept banner of silence as normal.

Rather than seeking out help, we feel like others will judge us or blame us, or tell us to get over it. So instead we stay silent. We suffer in isolation.

Because we stay silent, our pain grows until it is almost unbearable. Not only are we carrying the load of grief, but we also suffer loneliness, confusion and perhaps even despair.

We really do need to share our hurt in order to process our grief. Expressing the way we feel helps us to heal. Storytelling has long been proven to help us heal from trauma. Sharing what has happened helps us to understand it better (through having to form meaningful words about it).

When another person empathetically receives our story and reflects it back to us with their own words we feel validated and valued. All of this helps us to move on from the pain of it all.

Make time to grieve.

I found that after my losses I naturally wanted to do one of two things. I either threw myself into life and made sure every moment was busy with social catch-ups, work and kids. Or I wanted to hole up in my house, talk to no one and bury my head in books and Netflix (basically any reality that wasn't my own).

Which option is healthier?

I'd argue they were exactly the same.

Both of my reactions were forms of distraction. I was seeking anything other than having to actually deal with the pain of my grief.

Eventually though I realised how important it is to create time to tend to your wounds. Especially if you have other children who naturally provide an excellent 24/7 distraction from grief.

If you don't make time to deal with it, your grief will lay dormant until something triggers it, and then it will be as sharp and painful as if it happened just yesterday.

You might be tempted to rush straight back into regular life, perhaps taking on extra projects or tasks to distract you from your loss.

Distraction can be a helpful tool at times, to keep you moving in the right direction. But if you never allow yourself the space to slow down and feel it, you risk burying the grief and not ever truly dealing with it.

When we bury a trauma, our body naturally wants to heal it. Often we'll find situations keep coming up in our lives, triggering this same old pain bringing our attention to it so that we can finally heal it and move on.

Allow yourself to process the pain when you feel it rather than trying to bury it down and dealing with it later.

Making time to deal with your grief will look differently for everyone. Maybe you're reading this book because you intuitively know you need to do this but you're unsure where to start.

Create time each day to treat yourself with as much kindness as you can muster. It starts with just doing things that make you feel good. Activities that give you some space away from mental and physical distractions to process what's happened.

For me this time was working through my happy list, morning journalling, exercise, meditation, yoga, counselling, intuitive work, walking by myself, sitting on the beach, women's circles and writing.

For you, it could be any one of of these things - or none. Maybe you just need to allow yourself to have those big ugly cries when feelings come up. I can't give you a prescription for what will work for you (if only it were that easy) but I do recommend you find a way that allows you to feel your grief as it comes up while you continue to live your life.

Keep moving forward.

While constant busy-ness is unhelpful if we don't allow ourselves time to process and heal, so too is falling down the wallow hole. (Pretty sure that's not a real thing but it describes perfectly where you end up after a loss, yes?)

Don't get me wrong, there is definitely a time for wallowing, for truly allowing yourself to do nothing but feel. But you also eventually need to create a focus for your day - something to keep you moving forward with life, even when you don't feel like it. If you already have other children, they will be excellent at this. They will not allow you to wallow for long as their needs are completely oblivious to your grief.

If you feel like you may be spending too much time in self-pity you need to create something to keep forward momentum.

Take up a creative project.
Follow an interest.
Join a club.
Write your own happy list.

Do something, anything, that keeps you moving in a positive direction.

Admittedly at first it might just feel like you're 'going through the motions'. Eventually though you'll notice that you will start to care more about these things and the positive emotions you used to feel about everyday life will start to return.

Forgive yourself daily.

Some days you'll feel as if nothing has changed. You will feel normal and okay, like you can cope with life again. You may even forget your sadness for a little while.

This may be immediately followed by feelings of guilt, as if you have somehow abandoned your baby by not feeling the grief of their loss in every moment. Forgive yourself for this.

Other days you will fall apart. You will crash and burn and not know how to get out of the hole you're currently buried in. Life will feel too hard and not worth it. You'll feel like no one understands. Hold on tight on these days. Be kind to yourself. Forgive yourself for falling apart.

Some days you will take out your anger and sadness on other people. You might not even like who you are. Forgive yourself for this.

Don't beat yourself up over things you've already said and done. Do your best to apologise or just try and be a little kinder tomorrow, to others, and to yourself.

Forgive yourself daily.

Sharing the bad news.

In the early days after losing your baby, all conversations are difficult. I found once I'd explained the necessities of what happened I didn't really want to continue to talk about it any more, and quickly ran out of things to say.

Usually most of my conversations are future-related. I'm not alone in this. We as humans like to talk about what we're going to do, who we're going to see, and discuss plans for tomorrow, or on the weekend, or next year.

It's incredibly hard to talk to anyone after you've lost a baby because your future, the future that you've spent so long imagining, simply no longer exists.

The family dynamics you anticipated and the special occasions you planned to share with that extra little person are no longer going to happen.

You're no longer planning when your maternity leave will start and how you'll manage financially. You stop thinking about life in terms of before the baby comes and after the baby comes. You can no longer think about the holidays you were planning to fit around the birth of a new family member. Those purchases you planned to make, or did make, are now pointless. Your list of things to do before the baby arrives is now useless.

You are literally left with this great void where the life you'd planned used to be.

I think it's equally important to give yourself the time to avoid these awkward conversations, and then bolster yourself to push through them to get to the other side. The right timing of both of these options can only be known to you.

Of course everyone is different, but I personally found that in the first month or so I needed to become a hermit. I needed time to myself to process what had happened without having to verbally explain it to anyone else. At the same time though, being alone wasn't overly helpful either. I needed distraction from the intense pain of my loss but not conversation about it.

This is where your very best friends come in. Those who know what has happened and don't need to ask anything else. In the early days and weeks after losing a baby it's helpful for people to come over with something to watch or suggest an activity that allows you to be together, but that don't create awkward silences that inevitably feel like they need to be filled with conversation.

Eventually though, I wanted to start talking about it. Ironically I feel like this happened around the same time everyone stopped asking if I was okay and had moved on.

This is where either your partner or someone close to you who really understands your loss is needed.

It's also important to admit to yourself when this person can't be your partner. Their experience of loss is quite different to yours and while they too have lost a baby, their connection to the baby was also different to yours.

I don't say this to diminish their pain, but I think it is important to acknowledge that while we will never be able to truly feel and understand how our partners feel about the loss of a baby, they also never completely understand ours.

Sometimes a friend, or sister, or Aunt, or mother who has been through the loss of a baby might be a better person to talk to.

They *get it* in a way your partner can't. Sometimes, just feeling like someone truly understands and has felt the pain you're feeling can really help.

Eventually there will come a time where you need to gently push yourself past the hermit stage and re-enter life as you once knew it.

This might mean going through a few awkward conversations and scenarios. It might mean showing up to Mother's groups months later and explaining to almost strangers that you lost the baby. It might mean going back to that bbq and honestly answering the question *'So what have you been up to lately?'* and just having a few change of topic conversations starters ready in mind when the inevitable awkward silence begins.

I've found asking other people about their life always works well. People always want to talk about themselves, so deflecting to them will usually get them talking and give you a chance to pull yourself back together.

But do you know what? If you *do* break down in front of others, try not to sweat it. I think we would all be a lot healthier (and happier) if we allowed ourselves to be more honest about how we feel rather then trying to pretend we have it together all of the time.

I used to worry what people would think of me if I started bawling, so I would avoid social situations altogether. But once I pushed myself to go to a few, and inevitably did get upset, I realised that mostly people are just kind and lovely.

Even those who didn't know what to say really just wanted to try and comfort me. It was almost like they felt some of my pain along with me and in doing that, allowed me to let some of it go.

RELATIONSHIPS.

Share your grief

You need to be able to connect over the loss of your baby in order for you both to be able to move on as a couple, especially if another baby is on the cards.

After we lost our first baby, Andrew and I went on vastly different paths of grieving.

Initially we connected physically and emotionally. We cried together. We stayed close to home. We were both very tender and gentle with each other. This grief was very new sacred ground and we both tiptoed along it.

We also started trying for another baby very quickly after our first loss. (Too quickly in hindsight). The physical connection between us felt even more intense and trying again made this feel even stronger.

I guess trying again was a tangible thing we could do for each other to ease the pain. It was something positive we could do together.

We knew a new baby wouldn't solve our grief but we felt it was something we could actually *do* to move forwards in a positive way.

Ironically we gave no thought to the possibility that we would lose another. I literally never contemplated the idea that it would happen again.

Until it did.

Our second loss saw our paths of grief separate even further. This time we didn't discuss another baby. There was no shared excitement over the fact that we would overcome this sadness together by having another baby. We didn't do anything to prevent pregnancy but we weren't actively trying anymore either.

Looking back at this time I think we were both just really lost and bewildered by the whole experience. We'd lost hope. In many ways we just kept going through the motions of our lives together but we'd stopped truly connecting over anything.

He threw himself into the gym and work. I threw myself into my work and keeping busy with the kids.

We putted along like this for another 3 months, until we lost our third.

I grieved our third baby hard. I grieved harder this time because alongside the physical loss I was also grieving my desire to have a third baby. I had given up. We decided together that it was time for a break, perhaps temporarily, perhaps permanently.

I could no longer soften this grief by thinking of another baby. I needed to experience the void of possibly no future babies ever. When you've spent a lot of time dreaming of your future looking one way and it's completely taken away, it's bloody scary. My whole future felt meaningless and empty.

It's very hard to write this, especially when I have two other beautiful healthy children. I've experience criticism from others who have said *'But you already have two healthy children!'* (Perhaps you yourself have thought these words while you've been reading this book?)

I understand where this sentiment comes from. I get it. I really do. I get that these words come from a place of pain. I will never fully be able to understand what it is like to lose your first baby and come home to an empty house. In the same way that others will never fully understand what it is like to lose a baby after you've already had one. I'm not interested in getting into which is harder.

They're incomparable and equally horrible.

I do wonder sometimes how my boys will feel about the words I write here though, should they read them sometime in the future.

How can I explain to them that they are and were my everything and yet I felt for a while there that I wanted to give up. I guess I hope that they will understand the complexity of grief and know these two extremes, my utter devastation and my intense love for them sat together in my body, side by side.

Even though I felt incredibly lost and overwhelmed giving up on the idea of our third baby, it was entirely my love for my boys that kept me going. *They* were the reason I would get up every day and keep going. *They* were the reason I continued to laugh and love even when everything else felt dark and scary. *They* were my light and there aren't enough words in the world to describe how grateful I am to be their mother.

I remember feeling like Andrew didn't grieve our third baby at all. He did of course, but on the outside it appeared that he went on with life as if nothing had happened.

If you've already read Part One you'll know that eventually things between us came to a head and we had to get honest with ourselves and each other about how far we'd let things fall apart.

At that time these are the things we admitted to each other that we'd never really wanted to say out loud.

1. I felt like I loved these babies more than him (and therefore my pain was worse) because he didn't grieve in the same way I did.

2. I felt emotionally unsupported by him because he never showed me his emotions.

3. He thought he needed to hold it together in front of me, because he thought if he fell apart *we'd fall apart*.

4. I felt alone in my grief.

5. He felt alone in his grief.

6. I didn't really like who I was anymore (I was negative, lost and sad all the time).

7. I felt like he was using the gym and work as a way to escape me and our life because of how bad it was.

8. He was going to the gym because that was his way of feeling good about himself again.

At the end of our confessions it came down to:

1. I needed him to show me his emotions about losing our babies.

2. We needed a common positive goal or project to work towards together.

3. I needed to work on liking me and my life again (AKA watering the flowers of my life).

How to keep your relationship strong after losing babies.

Share with each other how you feel.

It may not come naturally for your partner to be able to speak about their feelings. And you may not feel like you have the energy to battle with them for their words.

Seeking support to help you communicate can be really helpful. Seeing a counsellor either individually or as a couple can help both of you find a middle ground in your grief. A third party, who is not emotionally involved will be able to ask the right questions to allow both of you to share openly and give each other empathy and understanding of your partners perspective.

Don't judge their experience of grief.

It's unlikely that their grief will look the same as yours. Forgive them for this. Losing a baby is not a grief that anyone can ever prepare for. It may feel hurtful that your partner doesn't grieve in the same way as you, but there is no roadmap for how this should look. What is important is that you can create the path to find your way back to each other.

Schedule time for you as a couple.

In the depths of grief it can seem unimaginable to even consider doing anything fun with your partner. Your entire future, your idea of what your future happiness looks like together as a family has been ripped apart. Connecting with your partner may even be physically painful, because all it does is remind you of who you no longer have and what you no longer have to look forward to.

Yes, this is incredibly hard but it's also a very important part of healing as a couple.

Start slow.

Watch a movie together, or your favourite show. This way you can be together without having to have conversations that are painful.

Build up to a walk around the block together, conversation may happen, or it may feel right that you walk in silence.

Eventually work your way back to a dinner date, or anything you used to enjoy doing together as a couple.

Schedule this time in weekly or fortnightly so that you can't back out or allow the busy-ness of life to take over. It is so easy to seek distraction when we are grieving, but what we really need is connection, even when it's painful at first.

Talk to your partner if you are feeling overwhelmed, especially as your date draws nearer.

I remember feeling a special breed of social anxiety after losing Orion. I would want to be my usual social self, but as soon as we were getting ready and walking out the door I would freeze. It was like my whole body was saying no.

A couple of times I backed out completely. Eventually though I opened up about my anxiety and found that just being honest about how I was feeling really helped.

Keep connecting physically.

Some women I've spoken to found their physical intimacy increased after losing a baby. Others found it difficult to even hug their partner, and would shy away from any sort of touch in case it led to sex.

I'm sure I don't need to tell you that physical connection is an important part of any relationship and even in the midst of grief, it can be a really important part of healing.

It helps to release hormones that make you feel good. When you're unable to find the words or actions to help your partner in any other way, intimacy can feel like one of the only positive things that you can share together.

Even just holding each other in bed before you fall asleep can help to reduce your anxiety. Extended physical contact helps us to calm our nervous system down and reduce stress hormones.

Also remember physical connection doesn't just mean sex. Sit on the couch next to each other and hold hands. Kiss. Touch each other on the shoulder as you go about your day. Let smalls acts of physical touch be reminders that you here, and that even when you're feeling sad, you are both in this together.

SUPPORTING OTHERS

"So often, we try to make other people feel better by minimising their pain, by telling them that it will get better (which it will) or that there are worse things in the world (which there are). But that's not what I actually needed. What I actually needed was for someone to tell me it hurt because it mattered." - John Green.

Let's be honest. Most people have no clue how to help someone who's lost a baby. They don't know what to say, and those who do say something will probably put their foot in it at some point.

They'll be awkward and uncomfortable in the face of your pain. They'll want to help, but they won't know where to start. I've lost three babies of my own and I still really struggle knowing the right words to say to help someone else through it.

Everyone who experiences this is different. Something that I would have appreciated, may be very different to what others want from their friends and family. So while I offer my suggestions here, these are simply some guidelines for how you might go about supporting someone who has lost a baby.

I will try not to focus entirely on the negative, but there really are some things that you should avoid saying and doing.

Please don't let this make you too afraid to say or do anything though. Saying the wrong awkward thing and being there, is actually better than saying nothing at all.

Personally I think it's probably best to approach the loss of a baby with the idea that there really there is nothing right to say. Nothing can fix this for them, and there is nothing you can do to make the pain of losing a baby go away. What you can do though is be a good friend, partner, mother, sister, etc (whatever your role may be).

You can show them that you care and love them, and that you understand how big this loss is to them. They need to feel this in the days and weeks after their loss but also in the months and years after as well.

The way you support them will of course change over time, but never expect that the period of grieving their baby has ended. Just like living children, we continue to have a relationship with the babies we lose for the rest of our lives.

They are always in our heart and on our minds and it helps us to feel that connection when others recognise important dates and memories as well.

Helpful things to say and do

"I'm sorry for your loss"

"I can't even begin to imagine how this feels, I'm sorry."

"I'm thinking of you and sending my love at this horrible time."

We want you to acknowledge our baby and our loss. We want to know that you know how bad this hurts (because somehow it makes it all feel a little less hopeless if someone else understands.) These words are helpful because they let us know that you care, without minimising our pain or trying to fix the unfixable.

"I've just dropped a casserole off on your front doorstep. I'll check back in a couple of days to see if you want visitors"

"I've just dropped a care package off at your door - wine, chocolate, tissues, blanket, and a little something to remember your little one by. Please know I'm here whenever you need."

While saying *'Let me know if there is anything I can do to help'* is good, just doing something is even better. Depending on your relationship you may want to also spend some time there with them as well, or maybe just do a drop and run a few times until they're ready to talk. Don't give up after the first few weeks. It can take many months before they're ready.

Other helpful things you could do:

- Deliver a meal once a week for a few months to their home.
- Invite them out to have coffee or lunch.
- Invite them to see a movie (no talking required and makes an excellent distraction.)
- Drop off groceries or a fruit / vegetable box at their door.
- Offer to watch their other children to give them time together.
- Deliver dessert to their door.
- Drop off a coffee on your way past.
- Deliver a flowering plant (or regular flowers).

"I've been there too and it was the most painful thing I've ever experienced. I'm so sorry this has happened to you. I'm here to talk or just listen if you feel like you want to."

"I'm so sorry. If you ever need a shoulder to cry on or feel the need to rage (I felt very angry after my losses) please know that I'm here."

If you've been through this experience too it can be helpful to share your story. Be careful not to make the sharing about your own grief though. Try not to share too much. Allow them to ask questions if they want to know more about your experience. Share that you've been through this as a way to let them know you understand how painful this is and that you're here for them if they need.

"Would you like me to take your kids for a couple of hours today so you and (partner's name) can have some time to yourself?"

"Would your two like to come have a playdate over at our place for a couple of hours this afternoon?"

While other children are often a great distraction from grief, sometimes we need to fall apart in our grief in order to heal. Offering grieving parents some time together by watching their kids for them is a really practical, helpful thing you can do.

"I just wanted to check in and see how you're doing. Sometimes it feels like it gets harder rather than easier, doesn't it."

"How are you feeling today? Want to catch up? Anything I can do?"

Initially when you lose a baby the offers of support and love are plentiful. After a few weeks and months it all seems to go quiet. This can often be the hardest time, as it feels like everyone else has forgotten your baby while you are still grieving hard.

Try to continue checking in and extending offers to catch up even if at first all offers are turned down. It really does help just to know that others are still thinking of you.

"Would you like help organising a ceremony to farewell your baby."

If you're very close to the parents or Mother who has lost, this can be a lovely way to show that you understand how big this loss is to them. Before 20 weeks, most couples won't have a funeral for their baby but a beautiful ceremony or ritual can be an important step in letting go and can help them feel some resolution in their loss.

Avoid (at all costs).

"At least you weren't further along."

"At least you were only 6 (or any other numbers of) weeks"

"At least it wasn't one of your older children."

These sort of statements hurt to hear because it feels like you are minimising our grief. It makes us feel like you think we shouldn't be feeling the immense pain that we're currently feeling. Try to avoid any statement that starts with 'at least'.

At least ... nothing!

There is no comparison you can draw here that will magically make us feel better about losing our baby. These statements don't feel like they come from a place of empathy or compassion. They come from a place of trying to fix things, and while I'm sure you mean well, these words really hurt. It isn't anyones job to fix this so please don't try to with these statements.

"You're still young you can have another."

"It just means there was something wrong with this baby, so it was a good thing they passed now. You'll have another baby soon."

"You'll be super fertile now."

"Well at least you know you can get pregnant"

Please don't start talking about another baby or pregnancy when we're in the midst of deep grief. You would never say to someone who has lost their grandfather - *'At least your other grandfather is still alive.'*

This baby was just as real to us as someone who we've known for many years. We've had a relationship with them from the moment we conceived, perhaps even before that. Our body and life has changed for them and we've planned our entire future around their existence. No other baby will ever be able to replace this one and while yes we may decide to start trying again soon, it will not be in order to replace the baby we lost. It will be to give him or her a sibling and to grow the family that we've always wanted.

"At least you have two other healthy children to focus on at this time."

Yes we may have other children, who are beautiful amazing gifts in their own right. But their presence doesn't lesson the pain of losing another.

Sure, I can admit children make excellent distractions from grief and can help to pull us out of it at times, but please don't suggest that having other children makes the pain of this any less. Our pain is real and horrible and the worst thing we've ever been through. Trying to make it sound anything less than that doesn't help us in any way.

"It was meant to be."

"Your baby is in a happier place now"

"It was God's plan."

"Time heals all wounds"

"Everything happens for a reason."

Just no. No one wants to hear this when they've just lost a baby. Over time, the pain changes. It becomes less unbearable, but it doesn't ever go away. Perhaps we may eventually be able to reconcile our grief and even come to agree with some of these statements in our own time. But we certainly don't need to hear them from anyone else.

When you're in the sharp pain of the first few weeks after losing a baby these sorts of statements can bring up immeasurable rage. If you don't want this anger directed at you, don't say stupid things like this.

"Yep I've been through that too."

"This happens to everyone it's not a big deal"

"Oh you'll make another one."

"Oh that happened to my sister's friend's Aunty. She ended up having a healthy baby the very next year."

Right now, we feel like our whole world has come crashing down. We're unsure how we'll ever feel okay ever again. Being told that our feelings are 'not a big deal' tells us two things.

1. You don't get it.

2. You don't care enough about us to try to understand our feelings.

Don't try to minimise our pain with these statements, especially telling us about your friend of a friend of a friend who went through the same experience.

Unless you are sharing the hurt on your own heart and what you went through, we don't want to hear about someone you know who has gone through this already.

"It probably happened because you were doing too much."

"See I told you that you needed to look after yourself better."

"Your body just needed to practice."

"Maybe it was because you did…"

Many of us go through a period of blaming ourselves, or at least questioning and trying to work out what we did wrong. We don't need you to reaffirm any of these fears for us. Stay away from any statements that sound like blame. There is no place for it here.

Advice from other women.

"Acknowledge the life lost, acknowledge the pain, be a shoulder to cry on without offering condolences and words of wisdom. Take care of them, let them sulk in bed, let them mourn and don't make them feel like they should be over the grief. The worst thing is still grieving and feeling like the whole world has already moved on and forgotten." - Amanda Pinter

"My coworkers were some of the most supportive people after my MC last year. They sent me chocolate covered strawberries, offered to bring me food, took care of my fourth graders and made sure I didn't make any plans for the days I took off. It was little things that made me feel supported like checking in during planning sessions. They never said anything cliche but just asked how I was feeling or if I needed a break. I think time is huge too and just acknowledgment of grief in general without saying the typical *'It'll happen when it's meant to be'* stuff. - Farren Francis

"The best support I had besides my husband was a friend who had also experienced a loss. She would message and check in every couple of days just to ask how I was feeling and if there was anything I needed."- Natalie Whalan

HEALING

"The moment that you start allowing yourself to feel is the moment you will start to heal."

Lessons from grief

Losing my babies has taught me more about myself than any other experience in my life. I am profoundly grateful for that.

It has taken me a long time to come to this place where I feel this way. It was definitely not how I felt immediately after losing any of my babies. Far from it.

If you're still in the *'This is fucked'* stage, then there is probably no way you will be able to accept the idea that some good can come after the death of your baby.

You will want to argue, *'But couldn't I learn this some other way? Why does my baby have to die for me to learn this, this isn't fair?!'*

I get it. I remember picking up a book shortly after losing Orion and when I read this very idea, I threw the book across the room and (maturely) stormed out. It pushed my buttons and made me fucking mad.

It also planted a little seed somewhere deep in my brain that said *'Perhaps there is something good that can come from this brokenness'.*

It definitely took a long time for this seed to sprout though. It was almost another two years before I was able to change my mind on this idea. But even in those early days of complete darkness it did give me some hope. It helped me to start looking for the light, for the lessons and for what would eventually be, making peace with it all.

Regardless of whether you can hear it right now or not, there is truth in this idea. There *are* lessons and gifts to be found in our most broken moments. During the darkest times in our lives our soul is being sifted and shifted. It can only come out of this process with new insight and wisdom.

I found it comforting to know that there were others who have been in this exact situation before me. It was helpful knowing that I was not alone in feeling like I wanted to turn and run away from it all, instead of facing the pain.

I think we all fight this. We want to move away from pain, to protect ourselves from anything uncomfortable. Yet we may need to be reminded that the only way to the light, and to the lessons on other side is to go through the fire. To feel the pain and to allow ourselves to experience all of it.

This is why I so strongly recommend giving yourself the time and space to sit with the pain and grief of losing your baby.

I want you too to be able to come out the other side of this experience and have gained something from it all.

I want you too to be able to find the meaning of your loss, for you. (Unfortunately this is an inside game, and no amount of looking anywhere outside of yourself for advice or meaning is going to be your truth.)

I can't even give you the answer here in this book. I wish I could. Only you can make this meaning for yourself. I can help give you some ideas and tools for how to start listening, but ultimately it is up to you. The only way to find the lessons of your loss is to get quiet and still enough to hear the truth that already exists somewhere within you.

Healing is a journey of feeling.

We live in a society of distraction. At any minute of any day we can plug ourselves in and numb ourselves out. There is no longer time for our minds to wander. We no longer have time alone with our thoughts while we are waiting in line, waiting for the bus or waiting for someone to call. Instead, we fill up all of these moments with instant distraction - social media, games, food, checking off something from our never-ending to do list.

In the early days after losing a baby, distraction is a god-send. It feels too painful to be alone with our thoughts and so we turn to distraction to numb the edge off our pain.

At first you may look to anything that will help you numb. Constant distraction; social media, binge watching episodes on Netflix, throwing yourself into work, that glass of wine at the end of every day. You become like a junkie, looking for anything to take the edge off the pain of your grief.

At first, numbing is what will get you through the days, when it is all too recent and painful. If you have other children being a little numb can help you hold it together for them.

Eventually as the initial shock of our grief starts to subside we may find that distraction is no longer our best-laid plan. We might believe that we can out-run our grief. We might even think by avoiding spaces and circumstances that give us time to feel the pain means we can somehow sidestep our grief altogether.

It feels easier to not have to face this pain head-on and so we avoid it. As time passes and the numbness continues we may even get to a point where we forget *how* to feel it.

We may think that because we no longer break down daily or that life has moved on so significantly that we have resolved our grief. But if we haven't allowed ourselves to truly feel it and allow it to release through us, we will always carry it with us. It will always be there buried deep down inside, ready to be triggered or played out in other areas in our lives.

It may show up in the way that we treat ourselves if we haven't resolved our feelings about our body.

It may play out in our relationships and make us fearful of getting too close.

It may be present in the way we mother our other children. This grief may make us fiercely protective to the point that our kids may feel smothered.

It may play out in the way we live our lives in general. We may be too fearful to take risks of any kind and instead play it safe in all areas to avoid further disappointment and loss.

Perhaps it shows up in the way we never sit still, and become addicted to work to avoid having time to think and feel.

Our grief may show up in any number of ways and the only thing that we can know for sure is that unless we allow ourselves to truly feel it, we won't be able to heal it.

This is not to say that the love and tenderness you feel for your baby will disappear too. It won't. You will always have a tender spot when you think of the baby you never got to keep.

However, you need to truly feel the pain of this trauma to release it's negative hold on you. Think of it like a physical wound that goes untreated. If you don't deal with it, it will fester and become infected spreading to other parts of your body (ie. your life).

If you can treat the pain, be conscious of it, and care for it well, in time it will eventually heal and what you will be left with is a scar. The reminder of the pain that was there and all of the learning you had to go through in order to heal yourself.

Create space to feel it.

The best advice I can give you to start healing from the loss of a baby is to give yourself the time and space to feel what you need to feel. This sounds ridiculously simple I know. Maybe even too simple. But I've found this to be true. It's both profoundly simple and simply profound.

How do you make space to feel?

I'm not sure what the answer will be for you. But I can share here what has worked for me and many of the other women who've reached out to me over the last three years.

Journalling - Writing down all the crazy in my head has been a really important part of my healing process. It helped me to understand my own jumbled, painful thoughts about losing my babies and helped me find clarity in my life again. In Part Four of this book I've included forty prompts to get you started if you'd like to try writing as therapy.

Meditation - You're either already sold on the idea of meditation or you think that it's not for you because your mind feels too busy and impossible to quiet. This is exactly the reason you need meditation.

If the rest of your life is jam packed, even just ten minutes per day will help give you the space to start hearing your own inner voice. (And by the way, she is different to that noisy negative chatterbox that is constantly rambling on in your head).

You may find at first that you break down and cry each time you try to meditate. That's perfectly okay. That's your body and your mind starting to shift the grief you've been holding.

If you've never meditated before I suggest starting with a guided meditation. It's easier to stay focused when you have someone else's voice guiding you. You can download the meditations included in Part 4 of this book at www.bettinarae.com/wateringtheflowers

Talk to a counsellor or a friend who understands - I can't even begin to tell you how valuable talking to a counsellor is after losing a baby. Counsellors are excellent at calling bullshit on the stories we tell ourselves. When we're hiding the truth from ourselves, they are able to show us where we need to reevaluate our thinking and beliefs.

Many times my counsellor has been able to pull apart the story I was telling myself about how amazingly I was coping to get to the heart of how I was really feeling. Without her support I don't think I would have been able to deal with my feelings after having multiple losses and I would probably still be sifting through the grief of it all today.

Allow yourself to fall apart. - We often think of healing from grief as 'pulling ourselves together' but I actually believe that falling apart is just as important in the process of healing. If you don't let yourself fall apart completely, I don't think you can pull yourself together properly. You will always carry a broken part of yourself that needs healing.

Don't buy into the idea that healing has to look clean and neat and socially acceptable. Bawl. Sleep for days. Pull it together one minute and cry into your breakfast the next. Do whatever you need to do to feel the extent of your pain, while also working with these other tools to slowly piece yourself back together.

Take a break from anything non-essential - I'm not suggesting you quit your job or do anything drastic, but where possible after losing a baby, give yourself the time to do as little as possible. You may feel compelled to stay busy to avoid having to feel but this is your survival instinct telling you to run away from anything that feels painful. And at this point, time alone with your own thoughts is bloody painful.

You need to spend time here to be able to move through your grief. Don't allow yourself to feel guilty for making time to do nothing but mope around the house and cry. Some days this is exactly what you need to do.

Mindfulness - Mindfulness is simply the practice of being aware, present and conscious. Like meditation this can feel incredibly painful when you're experiencing grief. When everything is so raw, your natural instinct can be to run and hide from it. Mindfulness can feel like opening yourself up to feel every excruciating detail.

Mindfully experiencing your grief simply means being fully aware of your experience. It means dealing with whatever emotions or thoughts that you feel with loving-kindness and compassion for your self.

It doesn't mean that you automatically approach grief with gratitude or that you try to be happy about what has happened (an impossible task to ask of anyone). But is does mean that instead of fighting against what has happened or questioning why, you start to observe your experience of grief so that you can start draw on the wisdom you need to get through it.

Mindfulness is simply the practice of opening yourself up to what is happening right here and now. We let go of the need to try and fix what is happening and instead just be within it.

Movement - When we experience a traumatic event we either do one of two things. We either process the trauma and feelings around it to let it go or we store the trauma somewhere in the body (Van Der Kolk, MD, 2014). We can carry around the emotions of trauma for months, years or even decades.

Grief can show up in the body as:

- tightening in the chest, throat, stomach
- aches and pains
- sleeplessness or lethargy
- oversensitivity
- shortness of breath
- no energy
- feeling weak
- feeling disorientated / unfocused

Sometimes we manage to bury our grief so far down that we don't even realise it's still with us until some new movement or exercise unlocks it from our body and suddenly we're crying or feeling really crappy for no apparent reason. This is why movement is a really important part of the grief process. It helps us to keep moving the emotions and trauma so that we can be free to let it go, rather than holding on and continuing to re-live it.

There is no right type of movement to release emotions or grief. For some, the intensity of running might be needed to shift stuck emotions and find mindful awareness. For others running might be just another form of distraction. They might be literally running from their grief.

As with all aspects of grieving, the movement that works for you is going to be completely individual. It could be yoga, dancing, walking, boxing, or something else entirely. Keep trying different options until you find which one works best for you.

Moving towards hope.

Losing a baby is an experience that changes you, there is no doubt about that. You cannot lose a baby without needing to completely rebuild yourself in order to come out the other side. There is no way that you can be exactly the same person after losing a baby. Sure, there are elements of that old you that remain. But as a whole, a transformation occurs.

Throughout this process we can either resist, or we can surrender.

We can stay stuck or we can choose to grow.

Life shattering experiences push us one of two ways. We either resist dealing with the pain of it all. We bury it down somewhere deep that we don't have to deal with it.

Or we can face the suffering head on and find ways to process it. This requires that we wake up to our own lives. It often means that we are forced to completely reevaluate our beliefs, the way we spend out time, our ideas about happiness and love.

We get to decide whether this experience wake us up from living an un-conscious life. Or whether it becomes what pushes us into unconsciousness and numbing to avoid the pain.

Suffering and trauma not only transform us but they also force us to answer the question *What matters most in my life?*

This can be an incredibly painful question to answer when you've lost a child, especially if your answer is 'children' or family, or your loved ones.

When you're in the depths of it, it can be hard to hear that good things actually do come out of the bad stuff. Or that you will feel happy again on the other side. But I can tell you that this is true. Even in the horror of it all there is light to be found.

Grief exposes us to our life in a way I'd never before experienced. It rocked me to my core and yet in a funny way made me realise how much about life I didn't know before. Life was suddenly split into two distinct time periods; before and after.

It completely changed my perspective. I mourned my naivety of before. That unbounded enthusiasm whenever I saw two pink lines on a pregnancy test, was no longer a guarantee of anything. If anything, now it meant the possibility of another loss.

Loss also makes you hypersensitive to all the losses of the world. It can feel like it turns up your empathy dial and suddenly you feel the pain of everyone right down deep in your bones. You imagine worst case scenarios everywhere. It sounds a little morbid, but it works to remind you that life is so precious, and that really all we have is now.

It can be a very long road from the loss of your baby to eventually coming to the place where you can assign your own meaning to the whole experience.

If you're reading this in the fresh pain of grief, you may want to skip over this section and come back to it later. I know because when I first heard that it was up to me to decide on what meaning I gave my three losses, I wanted to scream and hurl something at someone.

'What do you mean it's my decision?! How can this be so random and pointless and unfair and be up to me to simply decide what I want it to mean?!'

Now that I'm on the other side I know that they were speaking the truth. You may never find a scientific reason why, that part may always be unknown. But in the context of your whole life you will find a way to make meaning from the whole experience. Eventually you'll find yourself looking back on it and see that within the immense pain of it all there are some incredible gifts that you were given as well.

Presence. Humility. Empathy. Depth.

The experience of losing my babies changed my life like no other. While I would never wish this horrible experience on anyone, it's also something that I wouldn't now wish away either. Without these experiences my life wouldn't look the way it does now. I wouldn't feel the way I feel and my perspective would be completely different.

The biggest changes of all are probably barely detectable to anyone other than me. The way that I live my life now, minute by minute, rather than always looking ahead. This experience has completely changed how I feel about myself, my family and life overall.

It's ironic that the lesson of presence was given to me (again and again) given it's something that I've been reciting, *but not truly living* for the last ten years as a yoga teacher.

I have to admit, I'm pretty embarrassed to admit that to you. But I guess it's true that we're drawn to the things we really need learn the most.

Before losing my babies I felt like I was always searching, always looking for more (for what now I'm not entirely sure). I never felt like what I was doing was enough.

I was always looking for external validation in places where it didn't really even matter. Instead of where I should have been looking all along - in the eyes of my kids, my husband, family and close friends and of course most importantly, *within*.

Losing my babies floored me. It shook the foundations of everything that I was and did and made me realise how much of my life was actually inconsequential and meaningless. It also shone a big bright spotlight on how much of my time was wasted on people and places that weren't really important to me at all. It showed me what had really been most important to me all along.

I eventually got the message after our third loss and got rid of all of those things in my life that I realised weren't that important to me after all.

My approach to work changed completely. I realised that while I'd been so busy trying to create a business that I could do from home to be with my kids more, my two boys had been busy growing up.

Things had to change.

I let go of tasks that I didn't really enjoy but that I'd been holding onto because I felt a loyalty to those I worked for. I started saying yes to work only if it was important to me and/or helped us be able to enjoy life with our young family.

Losing my babies also completely changed how I approached my health. I had always been pretty healthy, but I realised how passive I was in my approach to my own wellness.

I would hand over my trust to doctors and other experts assuming that they knew best. I never questioned the fact that actually what they were all giving me all along were actually only opinions.

Throughout the pregnancies and losses my eyes were opened to the medical system and many of its failings. I realised that at the heart of it all, *I need* to be the number one advocate for my own health.

That means educating myself, seeking advice from doctors and alternative therapists but treating them all as merely options, rather than gospel. Above all I learnt to trust my own instincts on what I believe is right for me.

What I came to realise was that I needed to take my power back when it came to how I approached my health, especially around pregnancy. Instead of passively waiting for my acupuncturist, naturopath and doctor to tell me when I was ready to conceive a healthy baby, I realised that conceiving and growing a baby is *so much more* than just getting your physical ducks in a a row.

Physical health is definitely important, but I also believe that there is a mental and spiritual element to conceiving and growing a child. I realised only I could know when I was ready for all of it with my whole being.

In hindsight I can now see that after our first loss, I was not in a good place mentally. I was incredibly anxious and lost in my grief.

Each time I fell pregnant to the mental soundtrack of *'I can't lose this baby too.' 'What if I lose this baby, I won't be able to cope with another loss?'*.

I spent so many hours lost in thoughts of what losing another baby would look like, how I would cope, how I would tell people, instead of conserving my energy for actually growing my baby.

I don't think these thoughts are entirely responsible my consecutive losses but I certainly don't think they helped. I really do believe that we create our world with the thoughts we think. I do believe that keeping your thoughts focused on the positive outcome, does play a role in conception and growing a baby.

As I started to unravel my anxiety and realised how negative my thoughts had become I set about consciously changing them. I would write positive mantras every day in my journal and come back to them whenever I found myself slipping into the negative. *

A little note to those of you who find this book at the end of your trying-to-conceive journey. For those of you who have decided that your future doesn't include a biological child or maybe even a child at all. For those of you who are trying to find your way to go on living without the family you imagined. You can still use these same tools I used to find my way to acceptance, to find your way back to hope and to manifest a life that you want to live with or without a baby.

Oftentimes I would find myself repeating them silently to myself while I practiced yoga. They became my silent prayer to the universe.

They started as…

I am healthy and strong and so happy in my life. I have everything I could ever want.

When I felt ready they became…

I am healthy and strong and I am ready to conceive a healthy baby.

Once I fell pregnant they changed to …

*I am healthy and strong and I **am** growing a healthy baby.*

I would also take some time to write what I was 'calling in' each day. They were my intentions for how I wanted to feel and what I wanted to create in my life.

I wrote things like…

I'm calling in…

A sense of peace and contentment. The strength to accept my life exactly as it is right now. To be able to truly feel the joys of my life.

When I felt ready to try again they became…

I'm calling in…

The soul of our third healthy baby. We're ready to meet you and hold you in our arms.

The ability trust that my body is ready and able to carry and birth another baby.

A sense of calm to know that everything is as it's meant to be and that everything will happen in its own time.

When I fell pregnant they changed to…

I'm calling in…

The strength and calm to carry and birth our healthy baby.

I have to admit when I first started doing this it felt really strange, hopeless and a little bit silly. But as time went on, I started to notice that I was feeling negative and helpless less often, and more certain and sure of myself.

I began to feel ready to conceive another baby. Of course there were still doubts. Anxiety would creep in on occasion, but whenever that happened I just did my best to bring myself back to my positive mantras.

I also focused on the things in my life that *were* making me happy and did more of them. My happy list might seem like a really simple activity but it's really is powerful when you're stuck in a negative, anxious state.

Of course none of these things changed my outlook immediately and I think its unrealistic to expect that anything will be able to.

When it comes to grief - nothing happens quickly.

Transforming your feelings from guilt and hopelessness to acceptance and hope is a choice you're going to have to make day by day, moment by moment. Some days you'll feel like what you're doing is making no difference at all.

But after a couple of weeks and months you might notice that you're starting to feel a little lighter. You might realise that you haven't cried for a whole day or that you are naturally finding yourself focusing on positive things in your life again.

Don't expect an instant change, but also don't let that put you off practicing. One day you will turn around and you'll barely recognise the person you were before.

Surrender

I've always felt that motherhood is a role of pure surrender. It seems to be a reoccurring theme in my experience of it anyway. We have to give up control of when we'll conceive, give over our body entirely during pregnancy and trust that our body knows what to do during birth. Then in the early days with a new baby we're at the complete whim of an unreasonable wailing person who is unsure what they want, but very vocal in sharing how they feel about it.

Motherhood demands that you surrender your body, your career (or at least the version of it that you enjoyed pre-kids), your relationship, your friendships, your social life, your house, and the list goes on and on and on...

Don't get me wrong, I don't mean surrender in a necessarily negative way. I'm not saying these things are irrevocably ruined by becoming a mother. Just that motherhood requires that we let go of our control of these things.

Perhaps this is a life lesson not specific to motherhood; this understanding that we really have no control over anything, despite our desire to feel like we do. Maybe motherhood just speeds up this learning? It shoves it in our faces so that we have only two options.

Fight the changes. Fight against ourselves to feel like we have some control.

Or surrender to the way it all wants to unfold.

I knew all of this before I lost my babies. I'd fought against surrender for the first two years of motherhood. It almost ruined my relationship, my health and it stopped me from really enjoying being a Mum. I'd already surrendered to the regular stuff. I no longer sweated the lack of sleep. Our social life happened, or it didn't. We weathered the meltdowns and didn't stress over the small stuff of parenting anymore.

But losing my babies was the ultimate lesson in surrender. It was the BIG lesson in learning that really none of us have any control over the time we get in this life, or the time we get with those we love.

Losing a baby slams the reality in your face that this minute, right here and now, is really all we ever have. You can do all the planning you like for the future but the only choices you actually get to make are in the minute, the second, the millisecond. And in that millisecond the only real choice you have is over how you feel.

You can't choose what will happen around you. You can't control anyone else's behaviour, not even your child's (much as we like to think we can). You can't control the events of the day. But you can at any given moment control how you react and how you feel about the things that happen.

That's it.

The truth of this surrender is that our lives are made up entirely of the way we allow ourselves to think and react to what happens to us.

It can be a hard fact to swallow because as children we're taught the opposite. We are taught that we can control how our life turns out. We are taught to play by the rules, to work hard, to be kind and we'll be rewarded with a good life. But that's not actually the truth of it at all.

Life is going to present you with a series of events and it's our job to surrender to the lessons of it all. Some lessons we won't want to learn. Some will have to be presented to us three, or four, or five times before we finally crack and allow ourselves to think and react in a new way. It's why sometimes it feels like we repeat the same mistakes many times over before we can finally move on with our lives.

This is why a good, loving, kind, hard working person like you has been presented with this horrible experience of losing a child. Not because you've done anything wrong. Not because you're being punished. But because you are being asked, *or perhaps reminded,* that yet again life is about surrender.

You're being asked to get out of your head, to stop planning and trying to control where your life is going. You are being asked to live your life here in this present moment.

To love from this place here.

To be kind in this place here.

To make choices only from here - not from your feelings about the past or your fears about the future, but here - right in this moment.

To feel your emotions in this place.

To choose to be happy now.

I'm not going to lie. It's not an easy place to live and it's exactly why we spend so much of our time distracting ourselves with the past or the future. Right here and now is raw and unexposed. It is what it is and we can't hide behind the stories we tell ourselves about it.

But it is true and it is really all there is.

You're being asked to wake up and live and this truly is a gift. There is no greater shift in life than going from believing that you have control over where your future is headed to living truly in the moment instead.

Sure, it may sound like a trendy hippy catch phrase.

'Being in the moment'
'Staying present'
'Be here now.'

But actually isn't this how we used to live? We used to be deeply connected to the tasks we were doing in the actual moment, rather than constantly being somewhere else in our minds. Before the internet. Before smart phones. Before we all got so god damn busy trying to prove we're successful by documenting it for the world to see.

And yeah, I'm sure our grandparents still found their minds wandered to the past and present. I won't pretend this is an entirely modern phenomenon, but I definitely think we've made it a whole lot easier to live anywhere BUT the present moment.

Coming back to the present for me was like seeing my world for the first time again. I started delighting again in all of the amazingly simple things I get to enjoy in my life.

Things that I'd been completely missing because I was so caught up in having another baby, and even before that, in being seen as a good mother, successful at work, a great partner, etc. (The biggest irony of all is that I now realise I was already all of these things, I just hadn't realised it yet).

I started delighting in the hilarious personalities of my kids.

I felt immense pride in how caring and empathetic my two boys are, something I'd previously taken for granted.

I fell back in love with my husband and realised how lucky I am to have this man by my side who has changed and evolved with me over the last 10+ years.

I looked around our home and the beautiful neighbourhood we live in and realised how MUCH we already have.

I realised how much I value the work that I get to do.

I was missing all of these things before. I was so busy pushing, striving and hustling for my worth that I was missing all of these amazing blessings that I already had.

Reevaluating what was important, stripping back the stuff that I didn't really need to be doing and focusing daily on these gifts has completely changed how I feel about my life.

I can honestly look at my life and feel incredibly grateful for all of it now. And that's a really nice place to be.

To get here though I had to completely surrender to what I thought life should look like and instead learn to embrace what it actually looks like instead.

This isn't an easy thing to do and it's something that I have to constantly work at practicing. (Please don't think for a minute that I've found the secret and live here all the time. I'm constantly having to remind myself.)

We might fight the surrender at first. We might try to control everything about our fertility, to find THE THING that will fix our fertility issues. Or spend months searching for the answer for why it happened and why we lost our baby. Yet I honestly believe that we get the most from finding a way to surrender to our situation.

Control feels tight and heavy and hard and stressful. In comparison, surrender feels freeing and expansive. It opens you up to all the possibilities of life, rather than the hard work of trying to force life into a mould it will never fit.

In surrender we can stop being so busy trying to understand why and get back to living our lives.

Trying again.

After losing a baby some women want to jump straight back into trying-to-conceive whilst others could not bear the thought of losing another baby. Some may see the act of carrying a healthy baby to term to be a healing journey, while others cannot move past the loss to even consider future options.

Neither path is right or wrong.

It is important to be emotionally ready before you start trying to conceive a new baby. Yes I know, you'd like to know the specific date and time of when that would be.

We would all like a road-map for when life will finally start to feel better, a little bit brighter. Unfortunately it doesn't exist and there is no set point in the future that I can pinpoint for you as to when you will feel better and emotionally ready to conceive another baby.

I also don't know if there is anything you can do to speed up this process of healing from grief.

All I know is that you can either sit around thinking about healing or you can try a variety of different practices and rituals to ease the pain. At the very least it will help the time pass a little quicker than sitting around. So there is always that.

After we lost Orion I was adamant that I wanted to start trying again straight away. I knew that another baby would never be able to replace the one we'd lost, but I think in some way I thought being pregnant again would help me to start healing.

I was desperately looking for ways to feel better. I didn't know where to even start looking and so trying for another baby felt like the only positive thing that I could focus on.

Of course, life didn't follow the meticulously thought out plan I'd created in my head, and it was another 5 months before I would even see those two little lines on a stick. In the time between losing Orion and falling again I didn't do much, other than focusing on trying to get pregnant. To be honest I was pretty lost in it all, which wasn't healthy at all.

When I lost our second baby at ten weeks I remember feeling like '*Are you fucking kidding me?! How can this be happening again?!*' I was so shocked.

After our second loss I fell pregnant again in the very next cycle. I would tell people we weren't really trying this time, which is somewhat true. I was so lost in heartache that I hadn't actually thought about the possibility of conceiving again. But obviously we didn't use anything to prevent pregnancy either.

Losing our third baby really broke me. I could no longer see how or when I'd ever feel okay again.

It was at this point that I finally snapped and realised I needed to give myself a period of time without trying. We didn't set a certain number of months. One part of me thought it might be a permanent break. I knew that I needed to not think about conceiving or pregnancy or anything to do with babies in order to heal my heart properly.

This was honestly the best thing that I did.

It gave me the mental (and emotional) break I needed to properly deal with my feelings over the loss of our three babies and also helped me to start focusing on all the positive wonderful things I already had in my life.

I had done a little work towards healing prior to this but to be honest after giving up is when the real changes started to occur.

Not having another baby to look forward to, or think about, or plan for, left me with nothing to do but to stare at the wide gaping hole of grief in my life. It meant I finally had to deal with it. This break forced me to answer the question '*What if there is no other baby for us, ever.*'

I think this was a really important question for me to consider in order to heal. It meant that I had to start working on finding acceptance around the loss of my babies and create another way to feel hope in my life that didn't revolve around what I thought my family should look like.

I won't lie and tell you that I ever got to a place where I no longer cared whether I ever conceived and carried another healthy baby, or not, because that's simply not true.

My desire for another child always remained.

But I did find a way to feel happy and excited for our future and what possibilities were in store for us, *regardless of whether that involved a baby or not.*

It was only once I came to this place that I realised that I wanted to open myself up to all of it. I realised that if I wanted to carry another healthy baby I had to open myself up fully to this experience.

After losing Orion I went into the next two pregnancies already assuming the worst. It was like I thought I could protect my heart from the pain of loss by not being 'too invested' in these pregnancies. Which of course didn't work. Even when I tried to lessen the pain of losing a baby by pre-empting it, it still hurt as deeply as when I was naively optimistic about it all.

I decided if I was going to try again I was going to put my whole heart on the line. I was going to focus only on the positive healthy baby I wanted to create and not send out mixed messages to the universe.

I realised that all love comes with the cost of loss. You can't pick and choose which parts you get to feel. If you close off to avoid the pain of loss, you also close off from the possibility of love.

I decided I wanted to feel all of it. If the price of this great love was the possibility of loss, I was going to go all in.

Eventually I read somewhere *'What costs you more - fear or grief?'* and I realised that I was definitely ready to try again. I was ready to take the risk but be open and positive about it.

So where does this leave you?

I hope it leads you to realising that the only person who can answer the question *'When should you try again?'*, is **you.** Only you can know when you're ready to conceive another baby.

My only advice is to make sure that you're also doing the work to allow yourself to heal from your grief and not let trying to conceive become the only positive focus in your life. Keep living. Keep loving. Keep watering your flowers.

How long does healing take?

I'm not someone who copes very well in the negative. Does anyone though?

I'm not one to mope about and wallow. When I get knocked down I'm quickly dragging myself back up and asking *'Okay then, what's next?'*

I immediately start looking for a new plan, a new direction.

This is why after my first two losses I tried to throw myself into the 'new plan' as soon as possible. I tried to bandaid the hurt I was feeling with looking forward to the next thing.

But grief isn't something you can plan away. It isn't something you can get busy enough that you can forget about. It doesn't come with a map and there definitely isn't a timeline of how it should pan out.

We need to ban time limits on grief. Don't allow yourself to feel that you should be over it by now. Continuing to feel it many months and years later is a healthy experience of grief.

Big feelings come from a big love. You may find that the feelings for your baby and the hurt you feel when you think about losing them always stays with you and I think that's okay. I think it's unrealistic to think that the love and pain you feel for your baby will ever go away entirely.

For me, it really wasn't until I faced my grief that I felt like I was able to start moving forward with it. And I say 'with it' because I feel like it will always be something that I carry with me. In the early days I felt like it started to define me, which I hated. I felt like literally every minute of every day was affected by how heavy I felt in my heart.

These days though I feel like grief is one of the truest, softest parts of me, but it's not all of me. It's also not necessarily an unwelcome part. For me, it was about two years from our first loss to the point where I felt like I could talk about them without falling apart. I'm not sure if this is a short amount of time, or a long one, nor do I think it really matters.

Rather than wondering when you'll feel better or comparing your timeline to others, just keep moving forwards. Keep yourself open to feel. Learn the lessons of your great heartbreak. Ask for help when you feel like your emotions are too big for you to handle on your own. And keep working through your days taking each minute as it comes.

I can't tell you how long it will take, but only assure you that little by little; relief will eventually come.

Stress and anxiety of pregnancy after loss

A pregnancy after loss is entirely different to any pregnancy that came before it. I felt sad when I first realised that I would never again be able to naively enjoy pregnancy like I did with my first two boys.

During my two pregnancies I had after losing Orion, I was an anxious mess. For the ten weeks of both I literally felt like I was holding my breath and 'waiting to see' if this baby would 'stick'.

When I told people that I was pregnant I was almost dismissive of it. Like *'Oh I'm pregnant but you know my history so I'm trying not to get my hopes up and we'll just see.'*

I know why I was in self-protection mode but it's only in hindsight that I can see how negative that was for me.

I was perpetually experiencing and feeling the emotions of the worst case scenario because that's the image that played over and over in my head.

Here's the thing. Your body can't tell the difference between an experience you're actually having or one that you're only imagining. So basically my body was experiencing all of the emotions and stress of losing a baby before I even did.

It's also why I think it's so important to visualise and allow yourself to imagine (even if you have to fake it 'til you make it at first) the scenario that you actually want to play out. This is not just a woo woo manifestation theory. It's about physically creating the right emotional state in your body to carry a baby.

We have so much power over our minds, but so often we let them run on autopilot. We get so wrapped up in our anxious thoughts that we don't even realise that we can actually think other ones if we choose to.

But we can. And I think we have to during a pregnancy after loss.

At first I was practicing my visualisation every morning. Some days I could imagine a healthy pregnancy easily, other days I had to work a lot harder to keep the 'what ifs' at bay.

I wrote myself out a script (basically just a story of how I wanted it all to play out) for those days where I felt so anxious that I couldn't visualise a positive scenario. I would read it to myself to connect in with how I wanted to feel about being pregnant.

As the pregnancy progressed I needed this visualisation less and less, although if I was ever feeling particularly anxious I would come back it.

I also relied heavily on positive mantra when I found myself in a negative spiral of thoughts. I had a set mantra that I would repeat to myself whenever I found my internal dialogue going down the road of *'Oh my god what if there is something wrong with this baby too?!'*.

Whenever my mind crept into the negative I would repeat to myself *"I am strong and healthy and I am growing a healthy baby."*

Towards the end of my pregnancy when my anxiety became about something going wrong during birth my mantra changed to *"My body and baby are strong and we will birth with ease."*

I found that staying on top of my anxiety by looking after myself really well helped to manage it. However there were times when I let myself get too busy, or got lost in too much technology and stopped eating particularly well.

During these times I noticed that my general overwhelm and anxiety increased and so did my anxiety around the pregnancy. For this reason a pregnancy after a loss requires an even higher level of self care.

Try to figure out for yourself what triggers your anxiety and what helps to bring you down before you fall pregnant, so that way you have a toolkit ready for when you need it.

Triggers	How to manage
Being too busy, feeling like you have too much to do.	Prioritise. Write a list of everything that overwhelms you then circle only the absolutely necessary. Try and let everything else slide. Ask for help. Take a mental health day off work. Journal. Meditation.
Pregnancy & birth announcements	Take a social media detox. Unfriend those people who trigger you the most. Allow yourself to feel the shitty feelings and then go and do something that makes you feel good.
Ultrasounds	Talk about how you're feeling with someone who understands. Journal. Meditation.
Pregnancy tests	Track your cycle and only use them when you're actually late.
Getting your period	Take *one* day off to wallow. Give yourself this time and then pick yourself back up the next cycle. Practice cycle self-care (tuning in with your cycle and looking after yourself based on the different phases and energies)
Children / baby related events	Work on your boundaries. Learn to say *'No I can't come'* when you need to.

Special occasions - Christmas, Easter, etc	Create your own ritual for how you honour your babies on these special days. Eg. a special ornament, time to yourself, writing a letter to them. Journal how you feel. Gratitude practice. Eg. meditation, written list or share with loved ones.
Anniversaries - due dates, still birth and miscarriage dates	Make space on these days to feel however you need to feel and to honour your baby how you want to. Create a ritual of your own that helps you feel connected to them. Spend time alone. Reach out to others. Meditation Move your body to help shift emotions on these days.

PART FOUR - THE FIRST FORTY DAYS

Other than sadness the most overwhelming feeling I experienced after each of my losses was that of feeling lost. Trying to conceive, being pregnant and planning for a baby involves so much of our time and energy. You imagine what life will look like with a new little babe, how you'll manage your work and leave, how your relationship will change, and even when and where you'll take holidays. Losing your baby means that your entire future as you planned it is also ripped away from you. Suddenly all those plans are non-existent and you're left with this great big empty void that you're unsure how to fill.

This overwhelming feeling of being lost sent me seeking, although I wasn't entirely sure what I was looking for. I guess I was trying to find something, anything, to make me feel better and I looked everywhere. In distraction (both healthy and unhealthy - tv, food, drinking, working out, overworking), in people, in work, in treatments and healing, in yoga, in the stories of others, in books, online… everywhere.

Without a doubt though, self-reflection through journalling has been one of the most important practices for me in moving towards healing.

After reading about morning pages in the book The Artist's Way by Julie Cameron I started every day with writing. I found it really helped to give me the space to work through my grief (or whatever stuff I happened to need to deal with at that time) and to get 'the madness' out of my head and heart before my days filled with children and having to 'get on with it' started.

As I later discovered I was definitely on the right track. There are many studies that show that writing and sharing our stories is an important part in the process of coming to terms with trauma and healing from its effects (Lepore & Greenberg, 2002).

I have to admit though, some days convincing myself to pick up that pen and get started was incredibly hard. I would feel like I had nothing to write, or that I was just writing the very exact thing I wrote yesterday, so what was the point? I looked everywhere for journalling prompts that could help make those days where I felt resistant to writing easier, but I never found anything that was specific enough to my experience of grief.

So in the final part of this book I hope to share with you what I was looking for. Here you'll find 40 days of journalling prompts, healing practices and ideas that you can use to help you work through your feelings of grief and start leaning towards a place of healing.

Some days you'll find a simple journalling prompt, other days there will be an activity you might like to consider. Of course you will not wake up on the fortieth day and be over your grief. This is simply a place to start. These are practices and tools you can come back to at any time.

There is no right or wrong way to use them. You could religiously set time aside each day to focus on this healing work, or you could just pick it up on those days where you feel that you need some extra support.

You can work from day 1 to 40 in chronological order or you could just choose to do those prompts that call to you the most. Each day you could answer the prompt and then move straight into your day or let your words continue flowing onto the page and to where they need to take you.

Please let me stress here that there is no right or wrong way to grieve, or to work towards healing My goal in sharing these prompts and suggestions is simply to share with you some ideas for healing work.

I've been in that place of feeling lost and seeking. If that's you too, here is a place to start.

One. The very worst day.

"There is no greater agony than bearing an untold story
inside you." - Maya Angelou

It's hard to know where to start. I could ease you into this writing
process, but I want to be upfront about something right from the
start.

Writing is incredibly powerful in the healing process but it is by no
means easy.

Writing dredges up thoughts and emotions that you had buried
deep within you. It may feel dark and scary to look at these things
in the harsh light of words on a page but there really is no better
way to shift the heaviness of these emotions from your heart.

Let's start with what was likely the hardest part of your journey so
far. Share your story of the day/ days you lost your baby. You
might start with the moment you found out or knew that
something was wrong. If you gave birth, perhaps you describe the
moments that led to saying hello and goodbye all at the same time.

Can you describe this experience in as much detail as you
remember.

Who were you with?

What was your first reaction or feeling?

Where were you?

What thoughts flashed through your mind?

In that moment, what concerned you the most?

Two. A letter to your baby.

"Tears are words that need to be written." - Paulo Coelho

Our relationship with our babies doesn't end just because their short life has. Regardless of your beliefs about the afterlife or what happens when we die, you will always be the mother of this baby.

You are always entitled to feel both love and sadness for your baby.

There is no end to this relationship.

Today I'd like you to write a letter to your baby.

Perhaps you want to tell them what you miss?

Or maybe you'd prefer to tell them about their family and what you want them to know.

Let this letter be a way to honour the relationship that you'll always have with your baby and a way to channel the love that you continue to feel for them.

Three. Feeling it Meditation.

"The moment you accept what troubles you've been given, the door will open." - Rumi

Today we will explore where in your physical body you feel your emotions about your baby. Read the following meditation script (or head to my website to download the audio at www.bettinarae.com/wateringtheflowers).

Afterwards you may like to just sit quietly for a few moments to allow yourself time to process. Or you may feel drawn to write about how and where you felt your grief.

Find a comfortable seated or lying position. Let your hands rest comfortably and close down your eyes. Take a deep breath in and let your body start to become heavy and restful. Let yourself feel supported by the floor or chair beneath you. Allow yourself to sigh and relax into your position, letting go of any gripping or holding in the body. Notice that as you allow the body to relax there are certain parts of the body that want to continue to hold tension. See if you can breathe into these parts and soften them further on the exhale.

Rest in this simple awareness of the body, following the gentle rise and fall of your breath.

Start now to allow thoughts of your baby to enter your mind. You can choose what you think about. Perhaps happy moments, when you first found out you were expecting, or those harder moments of loss. Try to not let yourself become overwhelmed by a million and one thoughts all at once, but let them float slowly into your awareness one at a time.

Allow one thought to come to the forefront of your mind. Allow yourself to explore the thought a little. Perhaps imagining yourself going through an experience or having a conversation to someone about it.

As you let your mind explore keep your awareness on your body. Notice what emotions starts to rise in the body and where you feel them.

Perhaps there is a sick feeling in your belly? Maybe a tightness in your neck or chest. Or maybe there is an all-consuming feeling of sadness and you're unable to pinpoint where in the physical body this emotion is being held. That's okay too. Allow yourself to feel whatever is true for you. There is no right or wrong way to feel during this meditation.

Let this first thought that you've been exploring start to drift away.

Allow another thought to move into your focus. If the same thought wants to come back, allow it, it's simply asking to be examined some more.

Let your mind examine this thought. Let it play out in your head, all the while staying focused on the sensations that you are feeling in the body.

Breathe and let them go.

Start to allow specific thoughts to drift away now and stay focused instead on the physical sensations created in the body by your emotions. Allow yourself to feel these emotions fully. Try not to distract yourself by thinking of something else and resist the urge you may feel to end this meditation early to escape what might be intense emotionally.

Continue to breathe deeply as you allow yourself to feel whatever in your body is asking to be felt. If you feel like these emotions want to be released in someway simply let go and be guided by your body.

You may cry, sob, scream, laugh, shout, gasp. Whatever physical reaction is coming up for you allow it to be released. There is no reason to hold it in any longer.

Continue like this making sure you keep breathing deeply until you feel that the intensity of the emotion is starting to fade.

Allow yourself to rest just following your breath for a few minutes.

When you feel ready to, breathe some energy back into your body. Allow the breath to enter your body bringing with it a sense of lightness and ease. Stretch out in any way that feels good for you and slowly return your awareness to your physical position. Take your time slowly waking yourself up from this meditation.

Four. All the questions.

Losing a baby feels so unfair. It's so unimaginably cruel and inexplicable that you probably find yourself with a million unanswered questions each day.

Why did this happen?

What was wrong with my baby?

What is wrong with my body?

What did I do wrong?

How can I stop it happening again?

Why me?

Please know that it's completely normal to find yourself questioning everything and to cry out in anger and frustration at the lack of answers.

I think it's important to allow ourselves to wrestle with these questions for as long as we need if we're ever going to come to a place where we can find peace with or without the answers.

Write out all the questions you have about losing your baby.

Allow yourself to feel the full range of emotions around these questions. Anger, confusion, frustrations, disbelief, heartache.

Five. Mourn your imagined future.

"All the art of living lies in a fine mingling of letting go and holding on." - Havelock Ellis

When you lose a baby, you don't just lose them, you also lose the entire future that you imagined you'd spend with them. The dates you'd so carefully marked on your calendar. All of the milestones that you anticipated you'd celebrate. Their relationship with siblings (if you have other children). All of it.

It can be hard to explain to someone who hasn't been through the loss of a baby that a big part of mourning is letting go of the future that you imagined you'd share.

It's okay to ache for these shattered dreams. To feel angry that they've been taken from you. It's normal to feel lost and unsure now that you no longer have a clear picture of what's ahead. It's normal to feel like your whole life has come crashing down.

Write down all the plans and things you'd imagined for your life with this baby.

Allow yourself to feel fully the pain of all the things that will no longer happen because your baby is gone. Allow yourself to let go of the future you imagined.

Six. Grief is a manifestation of love.

"It seems to me, that if we love, we grieve. That's the deal. That's the pact. Grief and love are forever intertwined. Grief is the terrible reminder of the depths of our love and, like love, grief is non-negotiable. There is a vastness to grief that overwhelms our minuscule selves. We are tiny, trembling clusters of atoms subsumed within grief's awesome presence." - Nick Cave

Grief is our expression of love when that person is no longer physically present. Grief can only be felt where love once was. Try not to forget this as you move through all the stages of grief. Just like grief, the love you feel for your baby will always be with you.

Write about the ways that you can still show or feel this love for your baby.

Perhaps you can show it in the way you love the other children you already have or towards your partner. Maybe you can honour this love through the way that you look after yourself or through reminding yourself to live fully in each moment in honour of your baby.

Can you show your love through ritual and practice where you take a moment to connect with your baby before your start each day.

There are many ways to continue to feel the love you felt for your baby even after they're gone. At first you may feel incredibly sad trying to cultivate these feelings of love, but over time the grief will fade and your connection and love for your baby will remain forever strong.

Seven. Keep looking for the light.

"Hope is being able to see that there is light despite all the darkness." - Desmond Tutu

Even in our darkest moments there will be patches of light. It's important to keep looking for the light so that we don't feel completely overwhelmed by the heaviness of the dark.

Where is there still light in your life?

Where is there good still in your life?

You could list something as simple as an act of kindness you received recently, the feeling of sunlight on your skin, the taste of your favourite food or describe someone you love.

List all of the patches of light in your life.

Eight. Feel it.

"Grief can be the garden of compassion. If you keep your heart open through everything, your pain can become your greatest ally in your life's search for love and wisdom." - Rumi

Time alone does not heal all wounds, but a willingness to express and feel your pain over time will begin the healing process.

Give yourself permission to feel whatever it is you need to feel today. Whether that be utter sadness, despair, numbness, shock, disbelief, denial, anger....

Write it all out.

How do you feel today?

Try not to censor or edit yourself in any way.

Nine. Disconnect.

"I closed my eyes and spoke to you in a thousand silent ways."- Rumi

Some days you just need to switch it all off. Unplug.

Get out of the Facebook forums.

Stop scrolling Instagram and seeing the countless baby photos in your feed.

Put your feet in the grass (or dirt).

Watch the clouds.

Feel it. Breathe. Repeat *'I'm going to be okay.'*

How can you disconnect today?

Now close this book. Leave your phone at home. And just be.

Ten. Creative channeling.

"Should you shield the valleys from the windstorms, you would never see the beauty of their canyons." - Elisabeth Kubler-Ross.

I'd like to invite you to channel your emotions into something creative today.

You don't have to be an artist.

You could be sew something, put together a scrapbook or photo wall, write a letter or poem, make a piece of jewellery.

Choose something that you enjoy doing and that feels like a positive way to spend time with thoughts of your baby.

Let this project be something you can do with the love you have for them.

Eleven. Seek hope.

"Deep grief sometimes is almost like a specific location, a coordinate on a map of time. When you are standing in that forest of sorrow, you cannot imagine that you could ever find your way to a better place. But if someone can assure you that they themselves have stood in that same place, and now have moved on, sometimes this will bring hope." - Elizabeth Gilbert

Who can you talk to today who is further along this journey than you?

Reach out to them and ask for their support. Meet them for a coffee and a chat or just send an email with the questions you have on your heart.

Can't think of anyone?

My email inbox is always open -bettina@bettinarae.com

Twelve. Emptiness.

"The friend who can be silent with us in a moment of despair or confusion, who can stay with us in an hour of grief and bereavement, who can tolerate not knowing... not healing, not curing... that is your friend who cares." - Henri Nouwen

After losing a baby it is not uncommon to experience a profound feeling of emptiness in your life. There is a baby-sized hole in your body, in your life, in your heart.

It can be tempting to try and fill the emptiness with everything and anything - alcohol, food, work, exercise, relationships, etc.

Rather than trying to fill it, perhaps today you can just sit with and honour this space within yourself and your life. Honour the emptiness by filling yourself up with love.

Describe what the emptiness feels like to you.

How can you fill yourself up with love today?

How can you make yourself feel good without trying to fix the feeling of emptiness?

Thirteen. Get angry.

"It is impossible for you to go on as you were before, so you must go on as you never have." - Cheryl Strayed

Describe the anger that is present in your heart. As women, many of us have brought up to not show our anger.

We are taught that it is not feminine or appealing to show this side of ourselves. But just like all other emotions, anger needs to be expressed.

Underneath our anger we often find a whole lot of hurt. Unless we release the anger we can't even begin to deal with the hurt.

What are you angry about?

Let it all out.

Fourteen. Today I affirm.

Read the affirmation below and let it settle on your heart. Come back to it whenever you like you're struggling. You might even like to re-write today's affirmation into your own words so that it resonates more strongly with you.

"I deserve all of the self-care that I can muster. I am worth the time. I am worth the effort. I am worth the money. Today I will nurture all parts of me; the healthy and the good parts, as well as the broken and healing parts."

Fifteen. Denial.

"Denial helps us to pace our feelings of grief. There is a grace in denial. It is nature's way of letting in only as much as we can handle." - Elisabeth Kubler-Ross.

Describe your shock.

Where do you feel numb? Are there aspects of your grief that you are denying?

Sixteen. Just the next step.

"Even the darkest night will end and the sun will rise." - Victor Hugo.

After losing a baby it can feel overwhelming that all your plans for the future are gone. Remember you don't need to have all of the answers right now, you only need to be able to look to the very next step in front of you.

What's your next step? Keep it small.

Next minute. Next hour. Next day.

Little by little you'll begin to be able to see and plan a future for yourself again.

What will you do today to make yourself feel good?

What could you spend the next hour doing?

Seventeen. Love

"In all this world, there is no love for you like mine." - Maya Angelou

Describe your love.

Where is there love in your life?

Eighteen. Rest.

"Where you used to be there is a hole in the world, which I find myself constantly walking around in the daytime and falling in at night. I miss you like hell." - Edna St Vincent Millay

Grieving takes a lot of our energy. You may feel lethargic and sluggish. You might feel frustrated that you still don't feel like your old self. You might also be exhausted from keeping busy and trying to do all the things to avoid the pain.

Let yourself rest today, whatever that looks like for you.

Call in sick to work.
Ask a friend or hire a babysitter so that you can take the day to yourself.
Give yourself a break from your to do list and allow yourself to do nothing productive.
Let your focus be filling your own energy tank back up.
Go for a walk somewhere beautiful.
Sleep the day away.
Read in the sun.

Whatever makes you feel relaxed and recharged - do that today.

Nineteen. Letting go Meditation.

"The truth is, unless you let go, unless you forgive yourself, unless you forgive the situation, unless you realise that the situation is over, you cannot move forward." - Steve Maraboli

Today I want us to set the intention to start letting go. Just a little. I say 'set the intention' because this will be a process. You don't just decide and it is done. Each day, just a little bit more you'll be able to let go of your pain, your frustrations, your desperation and your anger. You'll be able to soften a little, live a bit more, feel a little bit more ease; even with the companion of grief.

Read the following meditation script or head to my website to download the audio www.bettinarae.com/wateringtheflowers.

Afterwards you may like to just sit quietly for a few moments to allow yourself time to process. Or you may feel drawn to write some reflections of your meditation.

Close your eyes as you take a deep breath in and allow yourself to settle into your position. You may sit or lie, whichever you feel like doing today. Lift your shoulders up towards your ears and then as you exhale them soften into a comfortable position.

Gently squeeze your belly in towards the spine and as you exhale let it be completely soft.

Engage the muscles of your legs, and then exhale and release your entire body into its position.

Notice a feeling heaviness in the body. A weight that pulls your body down onto the floor, or the bed or chair. Let yourself sink.

Give your physical body the permission to let go fully into the support beneath you. Allow yourself to rest here for a few breaths.

Start to notice any physical sensations in the body. In your mind's eye focus on any part of your body that isn't feeling good. It might be that you feel physical tension (like soreness in the shoulders), or it could be that you're noticing emotions in the body (like a sick feeling in the stomach). You may not know what you're feeling. Try not to get caught up analysing the sensation, just draw your attention to it.

As you breathe in I want you to imagine this part of your body expanding with the breath.

Breathe in for one, two, three, four, five.

Pause.

Breathe out for five, four, three, two, one.

Pause.

As you breathe out imagine any negative energy or tension leaving that part of your body.

Breathe in for one, two, three, four, five.

Pause. Imagine the area of your body expanding.

Breathe out for five, four, three, two, one.

Pause. Visualise yourself letting go of everything that doesn't feel good as you exhale.

Repeat this for the next five breaths, staying focused on this same area of your body.

Bring your awareness now to another part of your body that doesn't feel good. If you don't have a specific area you can focus on the area around your heart or your whole body.

Start by being curious about the sensations that you are feeling here. Try not to get too caught up in the words your mind wants to create about them, but try to allow yourself to feel without trying to distract yourself with other things.

Again as you breathe in imagine this part of your body expanding with the breath.

Breathe in for one, two, three, four, five.

Pause.

Breathe out for five, four, three, two, one. Let go of whatever you need to let go of.

Pause.

Breathe in for one, two, three, four, five.

Pause.

Breathe out for five, four, three, two, one.

Pause.

Repeat this for the next five breaths.

Slowly allow your breath to find its own rhythm again. Let your awareness settle now back into your whole body. Start becoming aware of the room around you. Notice any sounds that you can hear. Stretch your body out long when you feel ready to return and open your eyes once more.

Twenty. Permission.

"The holiest of holidays are those kept by ourselves in silence and apart: the secret anniversaries of the heart." - Henry Wadsworth Longfellow

There seems to be a lot of 'shoulds' around grief.

You should be over it by now.

You should grieve in this 12 step way.

You should be able to get back to your life by now.

You should be able to look on the bright side.

But the reality is, grief is as individual as you or I. As individual as every love. Just as there was no way to predict the loss of your baby, there is also no way to predict the journey of your grief. The only way to know what your grief looks like is to go through it.

Give your grief permission to look any way it needs to today. Let it show up where it needs to. Stop 'should-ing' all over yourself.

If you need to cry, let yourself bawl.
If you need to rage, rant and rave until you feel better.
If you need to sleep the day away, rest your head.
If you need to talk about it, pick up the phone.
If you need to write, let your words bleed onto the page.
If you need to fall apart, crumble.

Give yourself permission to grieve. But also give yourself permission to live. To love again. To find beauty and joy in your day even when your heart feels sad. Do it without guilt or shame that your grief doesn't look another way.

You have permission to feel it all. There is no right or wrong. There is no 'should' when it comes to grief.

Write about where you have been trying to fit your grief into what you think it should look like.

Twenty One. The Happy List.

"Nobody will protect you from your suffering. You can't cry it away or eat it away or starve it away or walk it away or punch it away or even therapy it away. It's just there, and you have to survive it. You have to endure it. You have to live through it and love it and move on and be better for it and run as far as you can in the direction of your best and happiest dreams across the bridge that was built by your own desire to heal." Cheryl Strayed

When you're in the muckiest depths of grief it can feel like there is no way out. You can't see a door or a window or even a splinter of light for all the darkness that surrounds you.

If that's where you are right now, writing a happy list may feel pointless, superficial and even just plain stupid. Maybe think of the list as laying the concrete foundations of your bridge to healing. It's definitely not the whole bridge and you've still got a lot of work to do. But it's a start.

Write a list of things that you can do that make you feel happy. Keep them small and simple. Choose things that you will do for no other reason than they make you feel good.

Read a good book in the morning sun.
Rearrange and decorate your bedroom.
Get a massage.
Stay up late chatting and having wine with your best girlfriends.
Go through your wardrobe and only keep what you love.
Do something new and fun.

There are no rules to the happy list. It will be as individual as you are. Once it's written, stick it somewhere you'll see it regularly. Try and work through it. Everyday if you can. At least one each week. Refer to it when you find yourself in the ugly depths of grief, desperately seeking something to make you feel better.

Find yourself again in your happy list.

Twenty Two. Comparison hurts.

"Comparison is the thief of joy." - Theodore Roosevelt

A funny thing happens when you lose a baby. (And by funny, I mean ironically terrible.) Everyone around you suddenly seems to be pregnant, or having a baby or living in a blissfully happy family bubble.

Except you.

You are back at square one. Maybe even lower than that. Square minus one... thousand.

It's easy to get caught up looking at everyone else and comparing your hell-hole to their happy family bliss. To believe that everyone else has it so much easier.

Where are you stuck comparing your life to others?

What comparisons do you need to drop?

Twenty three. Be here, right where you are.

"Be confused, it's where you will learn things. Be broken, it's where you begin to heal. Be frustrated, it's where you start to make more authentic decisions. Be sad, because if we are brave enough we can head our hearts wisdom through it. Be whatever you are right now. No more hiding. You are worthy, always." - S.C Lourie

We all experience grief in our own ways. Our stories are different but our heartbreak is shared. This experience is a place and time of darkness for sure, but I don't believe we're meant to stay in the darkness forever.

I also don't believe we're meant to hide and bury our pain. I believe our experiences, even our bad ones, are a wake up call. An invitation to feel and experience it all fully. To be present for the joy, the pain, the love, the happiness, the peace, all of it.

When you're in the thick of the grief, it doesn't feel this way. In fact, it really sucks. It feels unfair. It makes you angry.

Decide to just meet yourself right where you are. Right here.

If you're in the thick of it, be there. If you're starting to see the light, be there. If you've taken what feels like 20 steps backwards, be there too.

Where are you today? Describe it. Write it down.

Twenty Four. Today I affirm.

Read the affirmation below and let it settle on your heart. Come back to it whenever you feel alone or overwhelmed by opinions or lack of support from those around you.   You might even like to re-write today's affirmation into your own words so that it resonates more strongly with you.

"Today I release the need for everyone in my life to understand how I feel. I realise that when others say hurtful things, they are unintentional, and they simply have not experienced what I have. Rather than wasting my energy feeling angry at them, I choose to show them compassion for not understanding my grief. I choose compassion for myself and those I love in my life."

Twenty Five. Guilt.

"Guilt is perhaps the most painful companion to death." -
Elisabeth Kubler-Ross

When you lose a baby without explanation it's normal to look for
answers. To struggle to understand why this happened. Why you?
Why your baby?

Many of us blame ourselves. If only we'd eaten better. Rested
more. Relaxed. Remembered to take our prenatal vitamins. Stressed
less. If only we weren't overweight. Underweight. If only we hadn't
eaten that soft cheese. Had that glass of wine. Gone for that run.
The list is endless. And pointless.

If you continue to carry this guilt around with you it's going to eat
you alive. It's going to drag you down into shame and that's not a
fun place to be.

Give yourself the relief of letting go of the guilt. It's not serving
you and it's not going to bring your baby back either. Your baby
would not want you carrying this burden of grief for the rest of
your life.

As unimaginable as it seems, some things in life just happen for no
fucking rhyme or reason. This is one of them.

What guilt are you holding onto when you think about losing your
baby?

What lies are you still believing about the role you played?

What guilt are you letting go of today?

Twenty Six. Falling apart.

"There's a crazy lady living in your head. I hope you'll be comforted to hear you're not alone. Most of us have an invisible inner terrible someone who says all sorts of nutty stuff that has no basis in truth." - Cheryl Strayed

Sometimes the path of grief looks like three steps forward, two steps back.

Falling apart.

Putting yourself together again.

Breaking down.

Rebuilding.

What does falling apart look like for you?

What does letting the waves of grief crash into you feel like?

Describe a recent day where you let yourself fall apart.

Twenty Seven. Strength in numbers.

"Birds with broken wings often try to help each other fly." - Matt Baker

Losing your baby can be an incredibly isolating experience. We feel like we are the only one who has felt a pain as unimaginable as this. It's not the same for our partner. It's not the same for our mother.

It can feel like no one understands.

But I promise you there are others who get it. We are out here. You just need to find us. Other mothers who've felt the anguish of losing a little soul we'd wanted so much.

Mothers who've bled and cried and felt like they've wanted to give up. Mothers who've felt disbelief at their own misfortune, and rage at their own body's failures. Mothers who've felt your pain once, or many times over.

Allow yourself to reach out to others who have felt your pain. Hearing the story of another person who aches like you will help you feel a little less alone. It will help you know that you're not the only one who has had to live with this unbearable pain and show you that if they can survive it, you can too.

Twenty Eight. Laughter.

"Life would be tragic if it weren't funny." - Stephen Hawking.

Even in our darkest times there will be things that will make you laugh. You may clutch your belly and shake at something hilarious and at the same time wonder how you can laugh at a time like this.

What has made you laugh recently?

Has there been any ridiculously awkward and funny moments in the midst of your grief?

Twenty Nine. Gratitude

"Joy is the simplest form of gratitude." - Karl Barth.

Sometimes our memories can be stuck in depression, tainted by our grief. Sometimes moving on means finding a way to reframe our memories in a more positive light. It may mean finding a way to be grateful for the experience, even though it wasn't the one we wanted.

Are there parts of your experience that you can be grateful for?

Can you choose one memory and re-write it through the lens of gratitude?

Thirty. All of you.

"Allow beauty to shatter you regularly. The loveliest people are the ones who have been burnt and broken and torn at the seams yet still send their open hearts into the world to mend with love again, and again, and again. You must allow yourself to feel your life while you're in it." - Victoria Erickson

Your grief is one part of you, not all of you.

What does the rest of you look like, outside of of the parts that are mired with pain?

Where is there beauty?

Describe all of you.

Thirty One. Change.

"The reality is that you will grieve forever. You will not 'get over' the loss of a loved one; you will learn to live with it. You will heal and you will rebuild yourself around the loss you have suffered. You will be whole again but you will never be the same. Nor should you be the same nor would you want to." - Elisabeth Kubler-Ross

Losing your baby shatters you to the core. It breaks your heart. It rips apart the vision you held for your future. It throws everything you value up into the air like confetti and all you can do is watch it slowly float back to earth, observing which parts might come back to you.

At first it feels like the parts might never come back together. But little by little, day by day you will feel yourself start to return. A new you will evolve.

Today I'd like for you to reflect on all the ways that you've been changed by the loss of your baby.

What have you lost?

What have you let go of because you lost your baby?

Ideas? Beliefs? Roles? Relationships?

And what have you gained after the loss of your baby?

Strength? Understanding?

How have all the little pieces of you come back together in a new way?

Who are you now without your baby?

Thirty Two. Fear.

"No one ever told me that grief felt so like fear." C.S Lewis.

After I lost my baby I found that I was paralysed by the thought of losing someone else I cared about. I would feel sick and anxious whenever my boys got into a car with someone else, imagining every possible worse case scenario.

I couldn't bear my husband going away for work because I was always expecting the worst - a call that something terrible had happened to him.

Life suddenly felt incredibly fragile and like everyone around me might be gone in an instant. I was so afraid for everyone. But mostly for myself. I couldn't imagine having to bear the pain of another loss.

It wasn't until I realised that you can't live when you are bound by fear, that I started talking about them. When I kept quiet about my fears they grew and grew in the darkness. They were suffocating all the joy in my life.

What are you most afraid of after losing your baby?

Thirty Three. Relationships.

"The friend who can be silent with us in a moment of despair or confusion, who can stay with us in an hour of grief and bereavement, who can tolerate not knowing... not healing, healing, not curing... that is a friend who cares." - Henri Nouwen

Some people in your life will shy away from your grief. They will be awkward and uncomfortable in the face of your pain.

Others, perhaps surprisingly, will be there in your darkest moments holding space for you.

What have you learnt about those in your life after losing your baby?

Have you lost friendships?

Are some of your relationships stronger after your loss?

Thirty Four. Today I affirm

Read the affirmation below and let it settle on your heart. Come back to it whenever you are struggling. You might like to re-write today's affirmation into your own words so that it is more meaningful for you.

"I can feel my pain and anguish over losing my baby and still be okay. It is safe for me to feel. I allow myself to feel and to fall apart. When I'm ready I will pick myself back up and continue on."

Thirty Five. The light.

"I said: what about my eyes?
He said: Keep them on the road.

I said: What about my passion?
He said: Keep it burning.

I said: What about my heart?
He said: Tell me what you hold inside it?

I said: Pain and sorrow.
He said: Stay with it. The wound is the place where the Light enters you."

— Rumi

I remember my darkest of days. The pain was unbearable. I was angry and lost and wild. I would have done anything to have gone back to before I'd felt the searing pain of losing a baby.

Eventually though, I started to realise that it was my choice. I could either stay in this place of raging against my losses, of fighting the truth of them, of being bruised and broken by them.

Or I could find a way to surrender to them. To allow them to become a part of me, but not the definition of me.

From there, I started to see the light and the possibility of new things that can come from places of heartache.

At first it was only glimmers.

Tiny glimpses of good things that can come from loss.

Being able to offer true empathy to a friend going through the same thing.

The falling away of all of the things I used to stress about but that I'd realised no longer mattered.

Are you able to see any of the good that will come from your darkness?

Can you see glimmers of light in your own life?

Start looking.

Can you create it yourself?

Thirty Six. Your wild and precious life.

"Tell me, what is it you plan to do with your one wild and precious life?" - Mary Oliver

I know what it feels like to imagine you can't go on. That there is nothing left to live for and you may as well give up.

But while your heart is still beating (and you know it is because you likely feel the pain of loss there) you still have your one wild and precious life to live.

Rather than feeling like you can't live because your baby died. Continue to live *because* your baby didn't. Live a life that honours both of you. Live a life they'd be proud of.

Imagine when you meet again them saying to you *'I'm so proud of you for being strong when I left. I'm so proud of you for going on.'*

What does a life of your dreams look like?

What do you plan to do with your one wild and precious life?

Thirty Seven. Lessons.

"Experience: that most brutal of teachers. But you learn, my God do you learn." - CS Lewis

What was the biggest lesson you received from the experience of losing your baby?

What do you know now that you didn't know before? Good and bad.

(Try not to think too much about this question. Just write what is on your heart.)

Thirty Eight. Darkness.

"Only when we are brave enough to explore the darkness will we discover the infinite power of our light." - Brene Brown

Before I lost I really struggled with negative emotions. I didn't want to feel them. I didn't want to see other people struggling with them. Hell, I didn't even want to know they existed.

Grieving my babies taught me how important it is for us to feel the whole range of emotions - not just the positive ones.

If we don't know sadness - how will we feel the true joy of happiness?

If we don't know pain - we also don't know the true beauty of peace.

There is something truly freeing in knowing that. Feeling negative emotions is a part of life. When you realise this you can embrace all of it, rather than spending all of your energy trying to avoid the hard stuff.

This realisation has completely changed me. It changed my relationship with my husband. It's changed me as a friend, as a sister and a daughter. It's even changed the way I parent.

Are you afraid of feeling negative emotions?

How can you lean in to negative emotions a little bit more?

Write about all the negative emotions you've been feeling recently.

Thirty Nine. Re-write your story.

"Owning our story and loving ourselves through the process is the bravest thing we'll ever do." - Brene Brown

We're almost at the end of this healing project. At the very beginning I asked you to write your story.

I'd like for you to share your story again today.

Pretend you're telling someone you've never met before. Write whatever comes to mind without censoring yourself.

When you're done, look back and read your original version.

Has anything changed?

Do you share your story in a different way now?

Do you feel differently about your story in any way?

Forty. Meditation for hope.

"Hope begins in the dark, the stubborn hope that if you just show up and try to do the right thing, the dawn will come. You wait and watch and work: you don't give up." - Anne Lamott

Our final day together, when you're ready, is about cultivating hope.

It is my hope that during this meditation you can focus your mind towards the positive future that you'd like to create for yourself.

If you find that this practice difficult to do at first, please don't worry. Give yourself time. Eventually you'll be able to imagine a hopeful future again for yourself.

Read the following meditation script or head to my website to download the audio at www.bettinarae.com/wateringtheflowers.

Afterwards you may like to just sit quietly for a few moments to allow yourself time to process. Or you may feel drawn to write some reflections of your meditation.

Settle yourself in to a comfortable position. We'll start by taking a mental scan of the body to help our physical self relax.

Allow your body to start feeling heavy and soft. Notice the crown of the head. Imagine this part of your body softening with the exhale.

Release any tension you might be feeling in the forehead or temple. Let the cheeks soften and the bottom jaw melt. Let the tongue relax in the mouth.

Notice a softness flow down the neck to your shoulders as if a gentle weight was drawing your shoulders down away from your ears.

Relax into the upper back. Let the belly and mid back soften. Imagine a warmth through the lower back and legs. Softening, melting into your position. Notice that the legs and arms feel heavy now. Weighted to the floor. Allow yourself to feel comforted by this sensation. Maybe even a little sleepy.

The whole body is completely relaxed in its position now. Allow yourself to move your attention away from the physical body, knowing that you can leave it safely to rest.

Start to become aware of your thoughts. Are they present with my voice, or perhaps they're jumping around elsewhere, writing lists, analysing conversations you've had or will have. Maybe your mind is busy planning for possible worst-case-scenarios.

See if you can start to quieten the mind by focusing only on the breath.

Notice as you breathe in.

And notice as you breathe out.

Notice as you breathe in.

Notice as you breathe out.

Continue noticing the breath. Drawing the mind back gently to the breath each time it tries to wander off.

Start to allow the mind to rest somewhere in the future. You may pick a time a couple of years from now, or perhaps only couple of months or weeks. When you imagine is completely up to you. What you imagine is also up to you, but I'd like to suggest that you pick something that makes you feel good. Something that makes you feel hopeful and happy and like you can't wait to get there.

Imagine yourself living. What are you doing? What are you wearing? Who are you with? How do you feel?

Remember this visualisation is entirely up to you, so you are free to imagine anything you like. It can be as realistic or as dreamlike as you want.

Try to imagine your future in as much detail as you can. What can you smell? Taste? Hear? Feel? See?

Allow yourself to follow this visualisation in your mind's eye.

Stay here following the breath and visualising your positive future for as long as you can.

Slowly allow the vision of your future to fade, but see if you can keep some of the positive feelings that you created close to your heart.

Start to slowly breathe some energy back into your body. Move gently whenever you feel ready to do so.

Take the feelings of this meditation with you into the rest of your day and week. Whenever you need to tap back into feelings of hope, let this meditation be your salve.

CONCLUSION

I've tried to sit down and write this conclusion for days now. Every time, I find myself staring at the blinking cursor not knowing where to start.

I wish I had all the answers to heal your heart after losing a baby. I wish I had a magic trick or a pill you could take to make all your heartache go away. I know these are things I longed for when I was struggling the most.

But it doesn't work like that. And I hope after reading this book you're on your way to not wanting to wish it all away anyway.

Above all, what I really want you take away from this book is this.

Your baby is important.
Your love and grief for them is important.
Your heartache is important.
Your story is important.

And I believe sharing your story with others is important. It is an important part of your own healing and in many cases of theirs as well.

Now that you've allowed me to share my story with you, I would be honoured if you would share yours with me - bettina@bettinarae.com

REFERENCES

Stephan Lepore, and M.A Greenberg, "Mending broken hearts: Effects of expressive writing on mood, cognitive processing, social adjustment and health." Psychology and Health, 17 (2002)

Bessel Van Der Kolk, MD. "The Body Keeps The Score, Brain Mind and Body in the Healing of Trauma." Penguin Books (2014)

ABOUT THE AUTHOR

Bettina Rae is a yoga teacher and counsellor who has spent the last 8 years studying and working with women around fertility, pregnancy, birth and early motherhood. Bettina runs an online community where she share yoga and meditation practices with thousands of women all over the world.

Join her community www.bettinarae.com

Printed in Great Britain
by Amazon

31082365R00149